PRAISE FOR
THE EDGE EFFECT

"When I think 'brain,' I immediately think of my friend and colleague Dr. Eric Braverman. His new book is a must for practitioners, patients or anyone who wants to improve their brain health naturally. Finally we have a definite book that tells us exactly how to prevent and treat Alzheimer's, improve memory and concentration, treat and prevent anxiety and depression, and more."
—Dr. Shari Lieberman, nutrition scientist, exercise physiologist,
and author of *The Real Vitamin & Mineral Book*

"Health is care. We start with the brain and everything else will heal accordingly. Dr. Braverman has the key to this. This book is important for the planet to heal. Everyone with a brain must buy this book."
—Ben Vereen, actor

"Dr. Eric Braverman uniquely combines…a new and creative approach to medicine. Dr. Braverman teaches that brain health can be both monitored and measured and that such analysis is the key to unlocking every individual's health."
—David J. Steinberg, Ph.D, president,
Long Island University

"Dr. Braverman's…approach to the aging of the brain is unique. So much so that we have incorporated its message into our curriculum.…He is a rare doctor of great vision and insight."
—Ronald Klatz, M.D., president, American Academy of
Anti-Aging Medicine

"Dr. Braverman's connection of the brain's role in all illness, and in maintaining good health, is an outstanding contribution to medicine."
—Dr. Jay M. Holder, Laureate, Albert Schweitzer Prize in Medicine

"At a time when the U.S. population is aging…[Eric Braverman's] findings bode well as a valuable prognostic tool for brain impairment."
—Ernest P. Noble, Ph.D., M.D., Former Director of NIAAA
(division of NIH), Professor of Psychiatry, UCLA

"QEEG (BEAM mapping) is well accepted in the medical community and issued to assist diagnosis in medicine. It is an important objective measure of organic or physical brain dysfunction."
—Robert W. Thatcher, Ph.D., Professor of Neurology and Radiology,
Department of Veterans Affairs

The EDGE EFFECT

ACHIEVE TOTAL HEALTH AND LONGEVITY WITH THE BALANCED BRAIN ADVANTAGE

ERIC R. BRAVERMAN, M.D.

STERLING PUBLISHING CO., INC.
NEW YORK

Library of Congress Cataloging-in-Publication Data Available

12 14 16 18 20 19 17 15 13

Published in paperback in 2005 by Sterling Publishing Co., Inc.
387 Park Avenue South, New York, NY 10016
© 2004 by Eric Braverman, M.D.
Illustrations on pages XII, 4, 7, 9, 10, 11, 12, 13, 14 and 16
© 2004 by Sharon & Joel Harris / illustrationOnline.com
Illustrations on pages 219, 221, 223 and 225 © John Ueland
Distributed in Canada by Sterling Publishing
c/o Canadian Manda Group, 165 Dufferin Street,
Toronto, Ontario, Canada M6K 3H6
Distributed in the United Kingdom by GMC Distribution Services,
Castle Place, 166 High Street, Lewes, East Sussex, England BN7 1XU
Distributed in Australia by Capricorn Link (Australia) Pty. Ltd.
P.O. Box 704, Windsor, NSW 2756, Australia

Sterling ISBN-13: 978-1-4027-2247-9
ISBN-10: 1-4027-2247-8

For information about custom editions, special sales, premium and
corporate purchases, please contact Sterling Special Sales
Department at 800-805-5489 or specialsales@sterlingpub.com.

The programs described in this book are based on medical research and neuro-science, but they are not a substitute for personalized medical care and advice. Always consult with a qualified health-care professional in matters relating to your health, especially those that may require a diagnosis or immediate medical attention. If you are currently taking medication, consult with your physician regarding possible modification of this program to meet your specific needs.

This book concerns various medical issues relating to the brain, among which is Alzheimer's disease. This particular syndrome is very difficult to diagnose accurately. Although this book sometimes refers to Alzheimer's disease specifically, we are using this term to cover many forms of dementia or waning cognitive functionality.

CONTENTS

To my parents, Herman J. and Vivian Braverman, who raised me to appreciate the vital role of health and well-being in living an abundant life. And to my mentors, the late Clark Thorp Randt, M.D.; Carlton Fredericks, Ph.D.; Carl Pfeiffer, M.D., Ph.D.; and the late Robert Atkins, M.D. Without their guidance, brilliance, and innovative ideas, my own quest for total health medicine would not have been possible.

ACKNOWLEDGMENTS

FOR MY BELOVED wife, Dasha, who has been my inspiration, my love, and my comfort. Thank you for your enduring faith in me.

I am very grateful to my colleagues who have been invaluable supporters and insightful critics of my work, including Gary Null, Ph.D.; Tatiana Karikh, M.D.; and Alison Notaro, M.A. I also want to thank my mentor, Rodolfo Llinas, M.D., Ph.D., who taught me the value of the Edge Effect. I would also like to mention Kenneth Blum, Ph.D., my scientific father and co-author on fifty research papers; Nora Volkow, M.D.; Ernest P. Noble, Ph.D., M.D.; John Polich, Ph.D.; and Orrin Devinsky, M.D., who are all integral to my development as a scientist.

Many fine physicians and scientists have helped shape my work, including Vincent Giampapa, M.D.; Ron Klatz, M.D.; Robert Goldman, M.D.; Ed Lichten, M.D.; Denise Bruner, M.D.; Ron Rothenberg, M.D.; Michael Klentze, M.D.; Nash Boutros, M.D.; Robert Thatcher, Ph.D.; John Morgan, M.D.; Norman Sussman, M.D.; Titus Parker, M.D.; Daniel Amen, M.D.; Steven Sinatra, M.D.; Shari Lieberman, Ph.D.; Thierry Hertzog, M.D., and Oskar Varshavskiy, D.O. I thank them all for their invaluable contributions. I am also deeply indebted to Dasha Braverman, B.S., RPA-C, founder and director of the Rainbow Wellness Center, LLC, for her guidance, direction, and development of all the nutrional information regarding brain-healthy diets used in this book.

I am extraordinarily fortunate to have a gifted team of medical and administrative people who have helped translate my ideas into successful patient care: Paul Popkin; Ida Feit; Anish Bajaj, D.C.; Jackie DiMaria, RPA-C; Javier Carbajal; Eugene Perepada; Maja Kamber; Yelena Spivak, RPA-C; Yana Mazy, RPA-C; and Brad Bongiovanni, N.D. Your skills are unsurpassed.

I would also like to thank my staff members, whose loyalty and dedication to helping my patients cannot go unheralded: John Pillepich, M.S., Susan Kaplysh, Marta Kowalewska, Josephine Fileccia, Henry Weisberg, Volette Rodriguez, Dennis Kalevas, Xudong Fu, Tanya Perepada, and Aida Bicic. You have all contributed to making our practice, PATH Medical, what it is today.

I offer special thanks to everyone who has helped in the creation of this book. Special thanks to my agent, Carol Mann, for putting together such a great team. Bruce Scali, Robin Dellabough, and Peter Guzzardi were all important to refining the manuscript. Pam Liflander's unique literary skills and insight helped me bring my ideas to these pages. Deep gratitude goes to Steve Magnuson, who showed great faith in me, and to his many talented colleagues at Sterling Publishing, including Charles Nurnberg, Andrew Martin, Rick Willett, Ronni Stolzenberg, Karen Nelson, and Rena Kornbluh. And I will forever be indebted to Len Riggio. Len, thank you for giving me hope, inspiration, and guidance throughout the process of bringing this book to publication.

And finally, to my patients, the greatest teachers of all, for providing me with the material for writing this book—God bless you all!

INTRODUCTION

ONE OF THE indisputable facts of human anatomy is that the head is attached to the rest of the body. Yet, when the time comes to seek treatment for a medical condition or symptom, many doctors seem to forget all about the head, and the brain that it houses. I strongly believe that they are wrong.

Today scientists and doctors are just beginning to uncover the mysteries that lie deep within the brain, at a great new frontier of medical research. Medical care is finally moving away from the model of treating symptoms solely as they relate to individual organs and body systems and is beginning to look at the whole human body as one living system. In this holistic model every part is important, but the brain is king among kings.

As a doctor who has been focusing on brain research and treatment for more than twenty-five years, I know from firsthand experience that when your body is not working properly, the first place to look is your brain. The brain controls the body's health. Every day millions of people are diagnosed with a host of ailments ranging from headaches to insomnia, depression, obesity, heart disease, and even cancer without taking brain health into consideration. Yet in all but those rare cases where genetics is undeniably trump, your brain plays a critical role.

Twenty years ago, when I was a medical student poring over brain cells in petri dishes and researching the electrochemical nature of the brain, my work took place far off the beaten path, largely ignored by mainstream medicine. But today I'm marginalized no longer. Today a new generation of physicians and researchers is deeply involved in what I began to see back then: the brain holds the key to living a long, healthy, happy life.

The human brain is both exceedingly complex and remarkably simple. It has the power to send energy along billions of connections, evoking a sense of self that is capable at one moment of admiring the beauty of a rainbow and at the next of flying into a murderous rage. For years I've been presenting research papers on brain function as it relates to health to scientists, physicians, and scholars from around the world. Every year the size of these meetings increases exponentially, so I know interest is growing.

I've been passionate about brain research my entire medical career. When I was a medical student I was fortunate enough to meet Dr. Carl Pfeiffer, founder of the Princeton Brain Bio Center. Dr. Pfeiffer was a pioneer in his conviction that most psychiatric problems were caused not by emotional factors such as early childhood experiences but by brain chemicals. He proved that toxic metals could drastically affect the brain's chemistry, causing both mental and physical illness. I was so intrigued by Dr. Pfeiffer's research that I offered to join his team as his research assistant. Within a few weeks I knew that I would dedicate my life to exploring the role of brain chemistry in healing. I continued this work at Brandeis University and Harvard Medical School.

After earning my medical degree at New York University Medical School, I continued to study the brain at the Atkins Center and the Princeton Brain Bio Center. Dr. Pfeiffer had attributed some psychological complaints and hypertension to diet, based on brain-related nutritional studies conducted at the Bio Center. My interest piqued, I expanded on this line of inquiry, looking at conditions such as diabetes, obesity, and hypertension, as well as normal stages of maturation such as menopause, which contribute to so many other health problems.

During my medical training I realized that there was more to healing than conventional approaches. As I began to study Eastern medicine, I saw firsthand the healing abilities of herbs, and the power that the mind and the spirit could exert over the body. As I looked deeper into various traditional practices, I found more evidence of their effectiveness, and I became convinced that this softer approach had to be incorporated into a Western medical strategy.

By 1983 I had completed my formal medical education and train-ing and had studied widely in alternative medicine. I was determined to bring everything I had learned to bear on treating people, but I wasn't sure how all the pieces fit together. Every avenue I explored had merit, but each one seemed compartmentalized: the Bio Center concentrated on the brain to the exclusion of the rest of the body; natural remedies and a healthy lifestyle had demonstrable benefits, yet in cases of serious illness there was still a need for the high-powered interventions of con-ventional medicine. I found myself searching for a way to gather every-thing I had learned under the auspices of one universal schema that could serve as the basis for all medical care.

THE SCIENCE OF THE EDGE EFFECT

While I was searching for this grand solution, I met a celebrity who had recently undergone bypass surgery. As I listened to him, I realized that he wasn't getting his thoughts across as quickly as he used to on televi-sion; it seemed that his whole personality had slowed down. As an abstract matter, I knew that bypass surgery slowed brain speed by ten milliseconds. All of a sudden I realized that the man had lost his edge: his thinking was simply not as sharp as it once was, even though his medical problems seemed to stem from his heart, not his brain. This, I felt, might be the doorway to that elusive universal principle.

Looking deeper, I began to focus on the concepts that led to this book, ideas first brought to the medical forefront by Rodolfo Llinas, M.D., Ph.D., a world-renowned researcher of brain function and my mentor at NYU Medical School. Dr. Llinas was able to articulate a blue-print for the brain-mind-body connection, showing that brain biochem-ical imbalances could cause disease. He called this concept the Edge Effect. He also demonstrated how electricity in the human body reaches the brain and is processed through four biochemical neurotransmitters: dopamine, acetylcholine, GABA, and serotonin.

Today we know that good health requires that for any given body function, all four neurotransmitters must be processed in a specific order and in precise amounts. The Edge Effect amplifies small electrical imbalances into bigger health problems. The slightest deviation in the brain's activity can be felt in the body, and small electrical imbalances can become amplified into bigger health problems. Your brain chemistry can also become unbalanced when your brain is unable to process electrical cues correctly, which leads to one or more of the neurotransmitters becoming deficient. These deficiencies directly lead to decreased physical and mental health.

Dr. Llinas's groundbreaking research inspired me to approach his findings from a clinical perspective. While research scientists are always looking to understand why the body fails, as a doctor I'm looking first to heal, then to prevent illness, and ultimately to create abundant health over a long life span. To my mind, the Edge Effect could be viewed as having a full-spectrum impact. On one hand, it had become clear to me that biochemical deficiencies in the brain led to poor health. On the other, a balanced brain not only could restore you to good health but also was essential to maintaining a sound mind and body over the long haul. I had found the object of my search: a universal connection between mind and body, between the medicines of East and West.

I also believe that the Edge Effect can go even farther. If you enhance your brain chemistry, you can reach new personal heights. The Edge Effect can actually lead you into a state of physical and emotional bliss, where you reach a peaceful Zen mind, a power zone in your body, and a spiritual pinnacle for your soul. When you are at your physical and mental best, you are experiencing the positive side of the Edge Effect. This sharpness is the mark of a balanced brain that enables us to love others, remain calm, and effectively put our intelligence to its best possible use.

THE FOUR DOMAINS OF HEALTHY BRAIN FUNCTION

The Edge Effect can be used as a powerful tool to manage the four great domains of brain health: memory, attention, personality and temperament, and physical health.

One measure for memory and attention is the speed at which the brain processes information. This is influenced by all four neurotransmitters, but especially by acetylcholine. A normal brain processes a thought at a speed of 320 milliseconds, or roughly one third of a second. Each person's brain processes information much like the wave you might

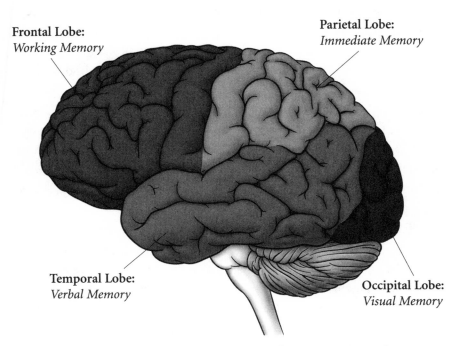

Frontal Lobe:
Working Memory

Parietal Lobe:
Immediate Memory

Temporal Lobe:
Verbal Memory

Occipital Lobe:
Visual Memory

The Four Lobes of Brain Function in the Memory Domain

participate in while sitting in the stands of a football or baseball game. In this analogy each person in the stadium represents a single cell in the brain. As he jumps to his feet and lifts his hands above his head, he passes the information along. If the timing is off, the wave in the stadium eventually breaks down. In your brain, if the cells cannot smoothly pass along information, brain speed slows, and your health and memory capacity begin to fade.

The difference between a resourceful mind and senility is only one hundred milliseconds of brain speed, which means you have fewer than a hundred milliseconds to lose over the course of your life. A human being reacts to light in fifty milliseconds, processes sound in one hundred milliseconds, and thinks in three hundred milliseconds. By the time our thinking is slowed to four hundred milliseconds, we can no longer process logical thoughts. When the brain slows down, which typically happens around the age of forty, we start to lose our edge. Unfortunately, while science has dramatically extended our life span in many cases, this gift will have little value if we can't think clearly or maintain our brain health.

A massive number of Americans are losing seven to ten milliseconds of brain speed per decade beginning at age forty. This sets in motion learning disabilities and neuropsychiatric problems as well as seemingly unrelated medical problems throughout the body. These medical, neurological, and psychiatric conditions related to loss of brain speed can cascade into obesity, anxiety, depression, psychosis, multiple sclerosis, and Parkinson's disease; 50 percent of Americans will have developed some degree of impairment from dementia or Alzheimer's disease by age eighty, and 80 percent will do so by ninety. Fortunately, most of these diseases are preventable once you learn to keep your brain in top condition.

Each of us has one dominant neurotransmitter. After taking the quiz in Chapter 3, you'll discover which neurotransmitter you are dominated by and where you may be deficient. By correcting these deficiencies and augmenting neurotransmitter production appropriately, you will naturally become a healthier and happier individual. Strong, lasting relationships will come to you more easily, and you will be able to improve every facet of your personal and professional life.

Since the majority of symptoms that cause us to seek medical attention involve a slowing of brain function or actual pauses in that function, the best way to fix the body and prevent disease is by addressing brain chemistry. If you already have a medical condition, you can stop it from worsening by restoring your brain health. For example, restoring deficient neurotransmitters to an unbalanced brain can revitalize other organs that are aging prematurely; left unchecked, their deterioration can lead to such varied conditions as diabetes, irritable bowel syndrome, gastrointestinal issues, sexual dysfunction and impotence, and even hypertension.

THE PATH MEDICAL APPROACH

Since the body functions in a holistic way, it makes sense to me that the best primary care should connect all types of treatment. About ten years ago I established a private medical practice called PATH Medical Services and Research Foundation—the Place for Achieving Total Health. I like to think of it as Eastern philosophy meeting Western technology on a new path to brain wellness. At PATH, we consider the whole body when formulating a treatment plan. We use established treatment protocols, both conventional and alternative, in tandem. By merging internal medicine and neuropsychology, this new form of medical care treats your brain, your mind, and your body as one entity.

My patients receive a definitive diagnosis, starting with a thorough examination of the brain, using the most advanced medical equipment. Over the past twenty years I have treated over ten thousand patients using my brain-based treatment protocol. I've watched patients with severe depression and problems with rage completely turn their lives around. Every day my office successfully treats common conditions such as insomnia, anxiety, exhaustion, infections, headache, high blood pressure, obesity, and attention deficit disorder. I have seen an Alzheimer's patient who couldn't even speak both recognize and greet me after consistent treatment. I've had patients close to death from cancer who have been helped by this brain-based approach.

My not-for-profit organization, the PATH Foundation, brings together nationally recognized medical experts to create a new agenda for public health. Our research confirms that brain electrical chemical imbalances contribute widely to the collapse of health. Americans currently spend more than $100 billion annually on neuropsychiatric problems, obesity, and Alzheimer's disease. The brain health checkups described in this book are vital to preventing brain chemical imbalances from destroying both the health of Americans and the besieged medical establishment that supports it.

BRAIN DOMINOES

The first step on the road to health is to recognize that you are in fact unwell. The body is known to react to many illnesses with a domino effect, where one small change can affect the workings of the entire body. In most instances, I see that first domino falling as a result of brain imbalance.

For example, a simple change in the brain chemical dopamine can cause your feelings of hostility and anger to increase. As your stress levels go up, your cardiac muscles strain and blood pressure increases as well. Eventually you become so wound up that you begin to burn up a second vital brain chemical, serotonin, which leads to insomnia. And when serotonin levels fall, your carbohydrate cravings go up: you eat more, you gain weight, and your kidneys begin to strain under the heavier workload. From this point, the downward spiral due to obesity takes over: your heart can become enlarged and your liver fatty, which can lead you down the path to a stroke, a heart attack, or even cancer.

Depending on which brain chemicals are affected, the direction of the domino chain can change. The common thread in all cases is that seemingly unrelated symptoms are actually caused by a brain chemical imbalance. To prevent the brain domino effect, to manage your symptoms so that you can effectively stop playing dominoes altogether, you need to balance your brain chemistry.

PROGRAMS FOR BRAIN HEALTH

This new book is an open door into my medical centers, so that everyone who reads it can benefit from our treatment programs and research. *The Edge Effect* is quite simply the brain's user manual, taking research into brain biochemistry out of the lab and placing it at your service in everyday life. By sharing what I've learned, I am handing you the secrets of the Edge Effect, which not only will make you feel better now but will also allow you to taste the ultimate in mental and physical health—an experience I call the Ultimate Edge. This goal is attainable for all of us.

First and foremost, this book is about prevention. You can keep your brain young and thriving by maintaining total body—and brain—health. Total brain health begins with a proper diet, an exercise program, and supplementation as needed. Prevention also means detecting problems early on by learning to recognize the earliest and most subtle shifts in the balance of your health.

The Edge Effect gives you all the tools you need to feel better, stay healthy, and identify the early symptoms of brain imbalance. This book is a straightforward guide to the anatomy, chemistry, electricity, and psychology that provide the building blocks of your day-to-day experience. You'll learn how your body functions and discover successful treatments that you can administer yourself. What's more, you can use this information to live better now.

In these pages I propose an alternative to the illness-, surgery-, and drug-based models of health care. Instead, you'll find a proactive, brain-based, early-assessment program that helps you avoid major health problems by treating minor ones. You will learn how to:

- Understand your unique strengths—and see how to reinforce them
- Identify your body's weaknesses—and discover how to improve them
- Monitor your health—and learn how to restore it

STRUCTURE OF THE BOOK

Part I focuses on identifying how the brain works, and why maintaining your edge is so important. You will learn about vital brain biochemicals and be able to ascertain whether your brain is balanced or unbalanced. More important, you will learn which of the four biotemperaments (which I call natures), based on your primary neurotransmitter, best describes you, and discover if you are experiencing any of the earliest warning signs that can lead to changes in your memory, attention, and mental or physical health.

Part II presents information specific to your own brain type. You'll discover how your brain chemistry creates the person you truly are and find specific recommendations for honing your edge through medications, hormones, diet, exercise, vitamins, and lifestyle changes based on your brain temperament. Finally, you will master the Edge Effect by selecting unique ways to relax, excite, or maintain your brain chemistry.

Part III addresses specific ailments in terms of brain health and matches them with likely treatments or solutions. In this section you will learn how to manage your current health issues and implement my recommended treatments while working with your own physicians. You will be armed with a program that will enhance your memory and attention by working within the context of your particular brain nature. You will also learn how you can bend your personality and improve your relationships with others simply by changing your biochemistry.

Everyone's brain gets a little out of kilter every now and then. With the tools in this book, you'll be able to get your health back on track. Once that's taken care of, you can begin to experience boundless joy and endless well-being in all aspects of your life.

PART I

UNDERSTANDING THE EDGE EFFECT

1
—

MEET YOUR BRAIN

IF ONE ORGAN differentiates humans from the rest of the natural world, it is the brain. Not so long ago intelligence was thought to be a factor of brain size. Elephants, thanks to ten-pound brains, were said to be so smart that they would "never forget." Birds, on the other hand, were thought to be less highly evolved because of their tiny brains (and we still disparage some people by calling them "birdbrains"). Now we know that humans have by far the most dynamic and highly evolved brain, even though it weighs a mere three pounds. Clearly, size doesn't matter.

It can also be said that brain function remains the most distinctively human quality. Almost all the other organs in the human body are replaceable and fixable, and often animals possess better versions of them. However, only in humans is the brain superior—which is all the more reason to put the Edge Effect to work by mastering the key to the health of our bodies and minds.

To truly understand how our bodies function and how to improve our capabilities, we need to start with an appreciation of how the brain works. Bear with me as we review the basics of brain function. The path to wellness begins with the smallest genes, which signal the brain to create chemical reactions that result in electricity traveling throughout your anatomy. Ultimately, your brain chemistry influences the four major domains of health: memory, attention, temperament and personality, and physical well-being.

3

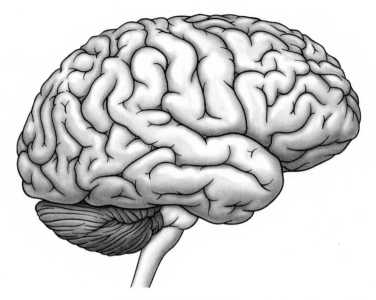

Right Side of the Brain

FROM GENES TO ELECTRICITY: DECODING THE BRAIN

For all that we humans tend to emphasize our differences, biologically speaking we are truly the same. The proof is in our DNA: the human genome sequence is more than 99.9 percent the same in all people. However, that 0.1 percent difference is all it takes for some of us to be healthy and others ill, some tall and others short, some quick-witted and others dull.

While DNA codes our behaviors and physical functions, it is not at the heart of what makes each of us unique. Our DNA is only as good as the transport system it creates for the transmission of information. That system relies on electricity. Just as you need a battery to start your car, the human body relies on electricity to stay alive. It is the literal spark of life, which energizes the body and creates our consciousness.

DEFINING THE EDGE EFFECT

Think of your brain as interfacing with your body, in much the way an electrical outlet functions inside the wall of your home. When you want to turn a light on, you plug in a lamp, and the electricity transfers from the house's circuitry into the lamp. In much the same way, the brain sends an electric current throughout your entire body, fueling your internal systems while maintaining your personality and orchestrating your health.

The connection between the outlet and the plug, or between the brain and the body, is one aspect of what I call the edge: it is the exact point where the brain and the body come together. When our edge fails, we fail. When it works, we function harmoniously. By mastering the Edge Effect, you can control the brain's signals to the rest of the body through changes in brain chemistry, intervening at the very place where brain information is transferred, ultimately allowing you to manage illness now and create abundant health later.

THE ELECTRICAL EDGE

The brain is the greatest generator of electricity within the body. We use four measurements to determine the relationship between brain function and the creation and delivery of human electricity to the rest of the body: voltage, speed, rhythm, and synchrony.

VOLTAGE

Voltage measures power, or the intensity with which the brain responds to a stimulus, which in turn affects the brain's ability to process that piece of information. This information can be cognitive as well as physical. For example, voltage determines your metabolism and the various states of consciousness, ranging from fully alert to deep sleep. Without proper voltage, you literally slow down and develop a dull edge to your actions as well as your personality.

SPEED

The brain's electricity runs through the body at sixty cycles or beats per second. Thinking occurs at two to three beats per second. The speed of your brain is based on how quickly these electrical signals are processed. This rate determines your brain's real or functional age, which might be very different from your chronological age. By increasing your brain speed you can improve memory, attention, IQ, and even behavior. When your brain speed slows, you can become forgetful and feel like you are losing your edge.

RHYTHM

A balanced brain creates and receives electricity in a smooth, even flow. By contrast, when electricity is generated in bursts, it is called arrhythmia, and it signifies the beginning of brain dysfunction. Rhythm determines how you handle life's stresses. When your rhythm is off, you might feel like you are getting edgy: this might make you feel anxious, nervous, or irritable.

SYNCHRONY

Electricity in the brain can be seen in the form of brain waves. There are four types of brain waves, each providing us with a level of physical as well as mental consciousness. The first type is called *beta,* which travels at a rate of twelve to sixteen cycles or pulses per second. When your brain is transmitting beta waves, you feel alert. The second type is called *alpha,* and travels at a rate of eight to twelve cycles or beats per second. When your brain is transmitting alpha waves, you feel creative. The next type, *theta* waves, travels at a rate of four to eight cycles or beats per second. When your brain is transmitting theta waves, you begin to feel drowsy. Last are *delta* waves, which travel at a rate of one to four beats per second. When your brain is transmitting a predominance of delta waves, you are at some level of sleep.

Whatever your state of consciousness, these four brain waves always appear in combination. Synchrony occurs when the four brain waves are balanced throughout the day. At night, our brain heals itself from the day's traumas by synchronizing the output of the four brain waves. If these brain waves are out of sync, then you might feel like you are going off the edge—you are not getting restful sleep, your mind wanders, and your personality is out of control.

IT ALL STARTS WITH A NEURON

The brain is able to coordinate your movements, control your breathing, and let you feel hunger, pain, sadness, and happiness through the electrical charges we've been discussing. However, this electricity is useless without the path on which it travels. Your brain activity begins with a stimulus: a thought, or input from any of the five senses. When the

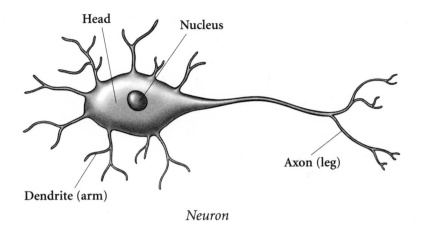

Head Nucleus

Axon (leg)

Dendrite (arm)

Neuron

information from this thought or your sensory nerves reaches your brain, your brain sends messages of its own down to the body. All of the signals going to and from your brain travel through your spinal cord. Together, the brain and spinal cord make up the central nervous system.

The smallest components of the nervous system are special cells called *neurons*. Each of us is born with one hundred billion neurons, and we continue to produce them throughout our lives. Every neuron has a nucleus, which contains the genetic material of the cell; dendrites, the branchlike extensions of the cell that receive messages; and the axon, a long extension that carries nerve impulses away from the body of the cell. Each neuron takes on a specific task, yet every neuron transmits information in the form of an electrical current.

Each neuron has thousands of dendrites that connect to other neurons to create your body's electrical network. Neurons come extremely close to one another but do not touch. The space between them is called a synaptic gap. Each of us has over one hundred trillion of these neuron-to-neuron gaps, or synapses. The axon of a neuron uses neurochemicals to cross this synapse and connect with the dendrite of another neuron. This connection is part of the circuitry of the brain, allowing that electricity to pass continuously through the neurons.

The flow of electricity is provided by the brain's biochemicals moving across the synapses to various receptor sites. These receptors are like fingers in a glove, each one fitting only one part of your hand. As specific pieces of these biochemicals lock into place, your brain directs how your body and mind function. The brain's biochemicals transfer electricity, which then sends energy and information to the rest of your body.

BIOCHEMICALS: THE BRAIN'S DELIVERY SERVICE

The brain and body function optimally when each neuron is correctly programmed to produce, send, and receive a specific biochemical. Each biochemical travels along a different path, resulting in a variety of physical processes. The free flow of these chemicals is the key to our well-being: if there is excess, the synapses become flooded and signals can't wade through to the next neuron; if there is a deficiency, the nerve signals might have nothing to travel on. Other parts of the body will react to these biochemical excesses and deficiencies by overworking or shutting down, leading to physical illness or mental instability.

The four primary biochemicals that define each of us are:
- Dopamine
- Acetylcholine
- GABA
- Serotonin

Together, these four chemicals make up the brain's code, much like the four base chemicals found in pairs on a DNA strand. Each biochemical creates unique electrical patterns that are transferred as brain waves. Studying individual brain waves and the relationship of brain waves to each other provides the information we need to explain the various physical and mental symptoms we experience, and then match them with a particular biochemical imbalance.

BRAIN STRUCTURE: ABOVE THE EDGE

Researchers have recently discovered that not only are these biochemicals and their resulting brain waves produced in specific locations within the brain, but they can also be found in the body, in such locations as the gut. These functional areas are connected to and complement each other. The brain itself is divided into three parts: the *cerebrum*, the *brain stem*, and the *cerebellum*. The cerebrum is further divided into two hemispheres, which are linked by a thick band of nerve fibers called the

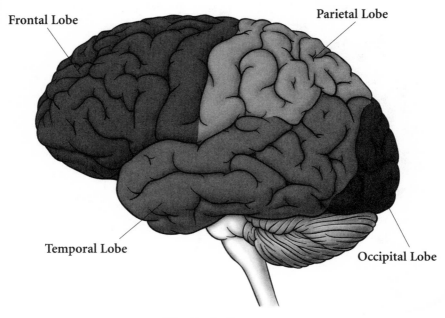

Frontal Lobe

Parietal Lobe

Temporal Lobe

Occipital Lobe

The Brain Structure

corpus callosum. Each hemisphere of the cerebrum is further divided into four areas called lobes; the cerebellum houses three lobes. Each lobe instructs our bodies to perform specific functions. With their help, we are able to think, reason, love, forgive, create, and remember. More importantly, these lobes, in conjunction with the brain stem, control automatic processes such as breathing and digesting. They affect our total health by managing all our internal systems.

THE CEREBRUM

The cerebrum is what most of us think of when we picture the brain. It consists of four pairs of lobes separated into two identical hemispheres. These lobes receive electrical currents from the nervous system and translate them into biochemical signals. Each pair of lobes is dominated by one of the four primary biochemicals. The lobes are also individually associated with one of the four measurements of electricity. The brain's electrical function as it processes biochemicals is the basis of brain health. The location of any biochemical surplus or deficiency is what ultimately controls your personality and your health.

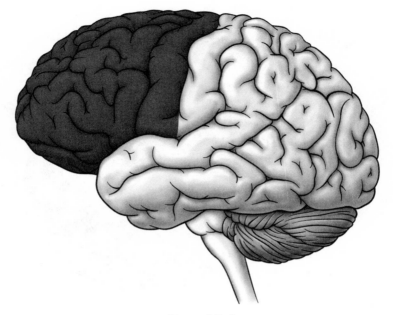

Frontal Lobe

Frontal Lobes

Every part of your body is connected through nerve cells that lead to the frontal lobes. Through these connections the body receives signals of sensation such as heat, cold, and touch. The frontal lobes control your movement and response to stimuli, and they shape your personality. Beta brain waves are created in the frontal lobes from neurons that produce the biochemical dopamine, which controls your electrical voltage.

Dopamine monitors your metabolism. It works like a natural amphetamine and controls your energy, excitement about new ideas, and motivation. Dopamine controls bodily functions related to power, including blood pressure, metabolism, and digestion. Dopamine generates the electricity that controls voluntary movement, intelligence, abstract thought, setting goals, long-term planning, and personality. The dopamine edge is characterized by its by-product, adrenaline. When you lose your dopamine edge, the physical effects can include addictive disorders, obesity, severe fatigue, and Parkinson's disease.

Parietal Lobes

The parietal lobes are the thought factory of the brain. Seated just behind the frontal lobes and on top of the temporal lobes, the parietal

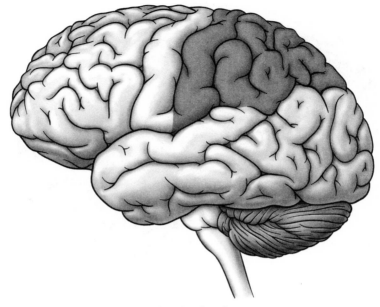

Parietal Lobe

lobes help the brain understand and react to sensory signals coming from your body. These lobes determine your brain's speed and relative brain age. The neurons here produce the biochemical acetylcholine and its associated alpha waves, which control brain speed. Acetylcholine is a lubricant, necessary to keep the internal structures of the body moist so that energy and information easily pass through each system. It is a building block for the body's insulation, called *myelin*, which surrounds the neurons throughout the nervous system. Just like the rubber surrounding electrical wires, acetylcholine keeps the signal from dissipating before it reaches its destination.

When your acetylcholine levels are balanced, you are creative and feel good about yourself. When acetylcholine is out of balance, negative effects can include language disorders and memory loss. Cognitive problems can run the gamut from childhood learning disabilities to Alzheimer's disease.

Temporal Lobes
Located just above the ears, the temporal lobes house the functions of memory and language. The neurons in these lobes produce the biochemical GABA and theta brain waves. These lobes assist in balancing

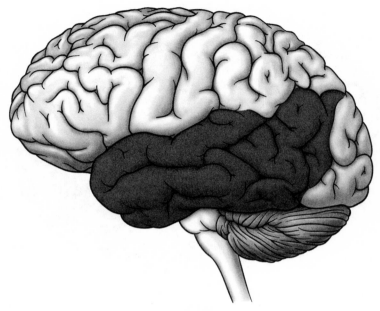

Temporal Lobe

the frontal lobes, which govern personality, and the parietal lobes, which control thinking and action.

GABA is the brain's natural Valium. This biochemical controls the brain's rhythm, so you function at a steady pace both physically and mentally. The GABA edge provides calmness to your body, mind, and spirit. GABA levels directly affect your personality. When the GABA edge is lost, physical effects can include headaches, hypertension, palpitations, seizures, a diminished sex drive, and disorders of the heart.

GABA is also involved in the production of endorphins, brain chemicals that create a feeling of well-being known as "runner's high." Endorphins are produced in the brain during physical movement, such as stretching, exercise, or even sexual intercourse. When endorphins are released, you experience the GABA quality of calmness. This release is often referred to as the Endorphin Effect.

Occipital Lobes
Occipital lobes can be found at the rear of the brain; they control the visual process. The occipital lobes also regulate your brain's ability to rest and resynchronize by producing the biochemical serotonin and its resulting

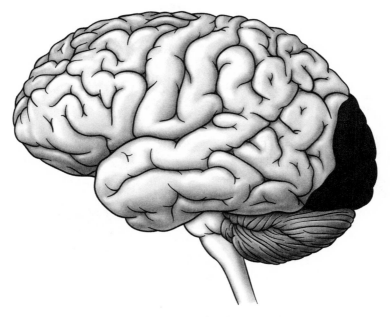

Occipital Lobe

delta waves. Serotonin provides a healing, nourishing, satisfied feeling to the brain and body. When your serotonin levels are appropriate, you can sleep deeply and peacefully, enjoy food, and think rationally. When the occipital lobes are damaged or out of balance, physical effects include depression, hormonal imbalances, PMS, sleep disorders, and eating disorders.

CORPUS CALLOSUM

This band of neuronal fibers provides the electrical connection between the right and left hemispheres of the brain, allowing the two sides to coordinate their tasks. The left brain controls the movements of the right side of your body, and the right brain controls the left side. There are also predominant behavioral characteristics related to each hemisphere, and each of us favors one side or the other. For example, left-brained individuals tend to focus on thinking, analysis, and accuracy. They tend to be introverted and rely strongly on their practical skills. The left-brained tend to be very disciplined and well organized and to see things in terms of parts or sequences. Left-brainers are GABA-dominant. GABA controls rhythm, and the classic left-brain type is consumed by making sure that everything is in good working order. They are

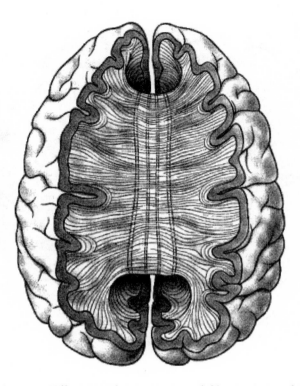

Corpus Callosum: The commissural fibers joining the brain's left and right hemispheres

concerned with traditional values and are blessed with common sense, thoroughness, and integrity.

Right-brained individuals focus on feelings, intuition, and aesthetics. While they are social and active, they prefer to direct their energy outward. They can be impulsive and spontaneous, and are usually more empathic, intuitive, and subjective. The right-brained person is dominated by the biochemical acetylcholine, which controls our creativity and speed. Right-brainers are famous for their buoyant and contagious enthusiasm. They are especially sensitive to the feelings of others.

The corpus callosum allows us to mix the best aspects of our left and right brains. For example, in dreams we creatively process our fantasies along with real day-to-day events. Fact and fiction merge, connecting the right brain's emotions with the left brain's processing of memory, uniting our consciousness.

FUNCTIONS GOVERNED BY THE LEFT HEMISPHERE

Deductive reasoning   Recognition of details
Logical thinking   Right side of the body
Practical analysis

DYSFUNCTIONS ASSOCIATED WITH THE LEFT HEMISPHERE

Dysgraphia   Right side motor impairment
Dyslexia   Verbal memory deficit
Impaired rhythm and singing
Language and mathematical
   impairment

FUNCTIONS GOVERNED BY THE RIGHT HEMISPHERE

Artistic vision   Left side of the body
Creative thinking   Understanding of the
Imagination   "big picture"
Intuition

DYSFUNCTIONS ASSOCIATED WITH THE RIGHT HEMISPHERE

Delusions   Neglect of hygiene
Denial of motor deficits   Spatial disorder
Dressing difficulties   Visual memory deficit
Left side motor impairment

THE BRAIN STEM: LOCATING THE EDGE EFFECT

The brain stem is the place where electricity is transferred between the brain and the body: it is where the Edge Effect takes place. The brain stem is the extension of the spinal cord into the brain, at a point called the *thalamus*. Using our earlier example, the brain stem is the two-pronged plug found at the end of a cord attached to a lamp. In this case each prong represents part of the autonomic nervous system. Between them these two prongs regulate all the involuntary and unconscious functions of the body, turning on and off all the organs of the body.

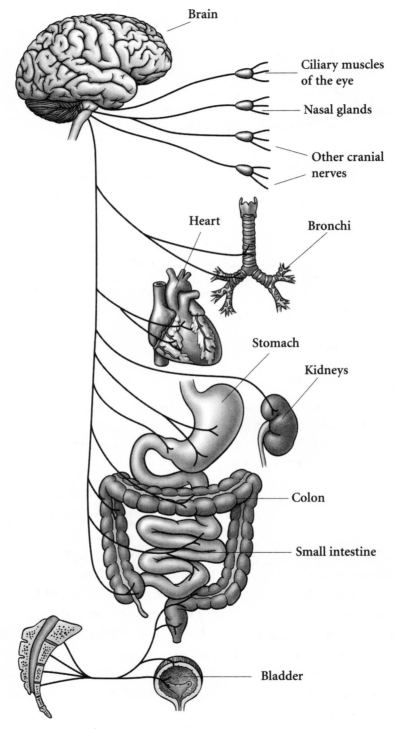

The Brain-Body Electrical System

THE CEREBELLUM

Located just below and behind the cerebrum, the cerebellum controls our balance and automatic movements such as arm and leg coordination. Animals with larger cerebellums than ours, such as cats, have incredible balancing ability.

THE OCEAN OF LIFE

A healthy brain and spinal cord float in a liquid called cerebrospinal fluid—what I call the ocean of life. Without it, the brain would dehydrate, shrink, harden, and eventually die.

The Edge Effect is also dependent on the ocean of life. In order to enhance its health and reach a higher state, the brain needs to continuously renew itself. When the Edge Effect occurs, your brain increases the production of essential biochemicals, and new neurons are created in the brain's center of higher intellectual function, the cerebral cortex. These new neurons can only be created in cerebrospinal fluid.

BIOCHEMISTRY FEEDS PHYSIOLOGY

All of us possess the same basic anatomy and approximately the same amount of proverbial gray matter. All of us sustain life with the same processes occurring within our remarkable brains. So why are we all so different? Why is one person more comfortable with a hammer in his hand, another with a calculator, and yet another with a clarinet? Why is one woman fulfilled as a nurse, another as a sculptor, and a third as the owner of a retail store? Why is one man thin and another overweight when they eat the same types and quantities of food? And why does each of us suffer from different health breakdowns at different times?

Again, the answers are found in the brain. Our genetic makeup individualizes each of us with our own biochemical deficiencies or surpluses. We are also dominated by dopamine, acetylcholine, GABA, or serotonin. These differences in brain chemistry translate directly into physical and behavioral tendencies. While we've discussed how the brain controls specific biological functions, its biochemistry also produces mental or behavioral characteristics. This is the biochemistry of personality.

TEMPERAMENT, TYPE,
AND PERSONALITY

Your temperament is the vehicle through which you express your emotions and values to others. Our brains process the four primary biochemicals in varying ways, and this combination determines our temperament and ultimately our personality. Before you can discover your temperament, you first need to recognize each of your individual preferences, or thinking styles. In the following categories, look at each pair and see which one best describes you:

Extroverts versus introverts

Extroverts direct their energy outward. They are very active and social, enjoy being in groups, and tend to talk before listening. They tend to be right-brain dominant. Introverted people require time for quiet reflection. Their need for privacy is especially important if their work is socially demanding or if they are under stress. Introverted individuals tightly control their thoughts, feelings, and needs, and may appear aloof or distant at times. They tend to be left-brain dominant.

Intuiting versus sensing

Intuitives focus on possibilities—always looking for new opportunities, new problems to solve, and new ways of doing things. They operate on their hunches, which makes them exciting companions. Their desire for change can put pressure on relationships if they fantasize aloud about how things could be better. They tend to be right-brain dominant.

Sensing types value accuracy in communication and prefer to base their statements on facts. They trust the tried-and-true ways of doing things and place a high value on tradition and experience. They live in the present and therefore become adept at managing the day-to-day details of living. They tend to be left-brain dominant.

Thinking versus feeling

Thinkers gather their information through logic and tend to

make decisions based on fairness. They are highly principled and often criticize others for not following the rules. Their seeming lack of empathy makes them come across as cold and overly blunt. They tend to be left-brain dominant.

Feelers have a warm, quick response to people and will try to say and do nice things. Feeling types want to be told explicitly that they are loved or cared for. Outside of relationships, they focus on process and human values instead of achieving goals. They tend to be right-brain dominant.

Judging versus perceiving

Judging people organize their outer world by means of structure, lists, and plans, and need closure when working on projects before moving on to something else. Their compulsion to organize and systematize comes at a cost to their ability to be flexible, be spontaneous, or accept change. They tend to be left-brain dominant.

Perceivers are curious people who love to experience new things. They tend to be spontaneous and flexible when it comes to organizing their outer world. They adapt quickly and tend to be interested in everything, which can cause them to start many projects but not complete them. They thrive on open-endedness. They tend to be right-brain dominant.

THE SCIENCE BEHIND
THE PREFERENCES

The PATH Foundation, working with other nationally recognized scientists, recently published research on the link between the brain biochemistry and temperament. The research clearly shows how each biochemical plays a unique role. We have found that dopamine accounts for extroversion and the preference for thought over feelings. GABA increases organizational skills. Serotonin is the generator of pleasure seeking and has been linked to various sensing and feeling behaviors that, if not kept under control, can lead to addictions. The implications of these findings are important to the rest of the body, in that each of the biochemicals also controls specific body functions. The table below identifies each personality type's most dominant and deficient biochemicals as well as the impact these have on the electrical functionality of the brain.

PERSONALITY TYPE	DOMINANT BIOCHEMICAL	ELECTRICAL FUNCTION
Extrovert	+ Dopamine	Increased voltage
Introvert	− Dopamine	Decreased voltage
Intuiting	+ Acetylcholine	Increased brain speed
Sensing	− Acetylcholine	Decreased brain speed
Judging	+ GABA	Increased calmness or rhythm
Perceiving	− GABA	Decreased calmness or rhythm
Feeling	+ Serotonin	Increased harmony
Thinking	− Serotonin	Decreased harmony

DETERMINING OUR BIOTEMPERAMENTS

Our temperaments are a combination of each of these preferences. For example, an intuitive individual is dominated by his style of decision making, but an intuitive thinker lives by thinking, while an intuitive feeler lives by feeling. Extroversion and introversion, except in the pure forms, are seen as modifiers of a person's temperament and are not a direct component of the four temperaments. Each of us falls into one of the following categories:

- Thinking intuitives are rationalists who are theory-oriented and skilled in long-range planning. They hunger for precision, especially in thought and language. They love power and have the ability to disregard criticism entirely. Their motto could be "Never take anything personally." Scientifically, thinking intuitives are driven by the frontal lobe biochemical dopamine and its associated beta brain waves, although other personality and biological factors can be considered. Thinking intuitives strive to be high-energy extroverts and might compensate for a sense of shyness with either caffeine or cigarettes (nicotine) to stimulate their personalities. Frequently a dopamine bio-temperament but other personality and biological factors alter the result.

- Intuitive feelers are idealists who strive to be authentic, benevolent, and empathetic; their greatest desire is to make the world a better place. Their motto could be "Always do your best." Intuitive feelers are regulated by the parietal lobe biochemical acetylcholine and its associated alpha brain waves, although other personality and biological factors can be considered. They strive to retain and create memorable events. Intuitive feelers may look for ways to alter their reality to make it more idealist or dreamlike by experimenting with illegal drugs such as LSD or PCP. These drugs tap into your dream state while you are still awake. Frequently an acetylcholine biotemperament but other personality and biological factors alter the result.

- Organization and tradition dominate sensing judging temperaments. Sensitive judging people can be described as guardians and are skilled at ensuring that everything is in the right place at the right time; they look to the past and tradition, and regard their duty as preserving conventional values. Relationships are of utmost importance to them. Their motto could be "Always keep your word." Sensitive judging people are often governed by the temporal lobe biochemical GABA and its associated theta brain waves, although other personality and biological factors can be considered. Sensitive judgers try to remain calm. They might use alcohol as a way of quieting their compulsiveness. Frequently a GABA biotemperament but other personality and biological factors alter the result.

- Sensitive perceivers are artisans who act on impulse and seek adventure and experience; they are often drawn to the manual and performing arts. They prize nothing more than fun. Their motto could be "Live through experience." Sensitive perceivers are ruled by the occipital lobe biochemical serotonin and its associated delta brain waves, although other personality and biological factors can be considered. Sensitive perceivers are driven by their moods. They often choose foods that they know will affect their moods, such as doughnuts or other carbohydrate-rich desserts, which will make them feel satisfied, if only temporarily. Frequently a serotonin biotemperament but other personality and biological factors alter the result.

PERSONALITY GOVERNED BY BIOCHEMISTRY

Temperaments become more complex as you include additional preferences from each category that are dominated by other biochemicals. The individual combinations directly determine our overall personality or type. While temperament is governed by a specific biochemical, it is the individualized combination of the four primary neurotransmitters that determines each personality.

When our biochemicals are balanced, our behavior stays within a healthy range. When there are excesses, severe psychiatric conditions can occur. When there are deficiencies, less serious antisocial behavior develops. Disturbances in our personality and emotional life are imbalances in our biotemperment. The good news is that the Edge Effect heals these imbalances. We all exhibit low moments in our personalities, and it is interesting to see which biochemicals influence specific "bad" behaviors.

Dopamine-deficient personality

The loner. When balanced, this person is organized, neat, frugal, and no trouble to others. When out of balance, this person lacks the energy to socialize and appears to lose the feelings of love, joy, sadness, desire, or rage. A natural remoteness becomes extreme by total avoidance of social interaction.

The procrastinator. When balanced, this person is flexible, giving, accommodating, available, and willing to go the extra mile for a friend. Out of balance, this person lacks the energy to finish any assignment or task. A procrastinator avoids meeting deadlines and deliberately works slowly on unappealing tasks. If angry, a procrastinator will avoid confrontation.

Acetylcholine-deficient personality

The eccentric. Normally the eccentric keeps to himself. At worst, the absence of thought connections to people and the world makes the eccentric's behavior seem odd, even bizarre. This personality feels normal in isolated situations and steers away from human interaction. The eccentric lives in a dream world consisting of magical behavior and wild visions, although outwardly he appears colorless and inexpressive. When even mildly stressed, an eccentric can easily become a danger to himself and others.

The perfectionist. Normally this profile is hardworking, detail-oriented, devoted, and exacting. Perfectionism and self-discipline are the hallmarks of this personality type—qualities that can be pluses or minuses depending on the extent of brain imbalance. Perfectionism can make someone an excellent worker, but it can also interfere with decision making, since striving for the ideal in everything is simply not realistic. Self-discipline gives the perfectionist's life structure but can also produce a rigidity that makes her unapproachable. The perfectionist is a classic workaholic who retains tight self-control at the expense of relaxation, enjoyment, and warmth. The perfectionist lacks the ability to end a project or get off task.

GABA-deficient personality
The unstable personality. In balance, this person meets the needs of others. Unbalanced, this type can lack control in every aspect of life: mood, relationships, identity, and impulses. Emotions are mercurial and without boundaries, moving rapidly from love to hate, from happiness to rage. Personal care is neglected, and a general feeling of emptiness persists as a result of loss of sustained relationships.

The drama queen. This person is a catalyst for creating change, growth, and development of self and others. When out of balance, the drama queen is inappropriately theatrical, loving and living for the big moment, which seems to be present every day. This person has a wild streak and often insists on being the center of attention, constantly searching for reassurance of his worth. He becomes totally disinterested in others' needs and ideas, even though social interaction is vital. The dramatic personality lacks boundaries between self and society, so that all of such a person's daily problems become everyone's concern.

Serotonin-deficient personality

The self-absorbed personality. Normally this person is a high achiever. However, when unbalanced, the self-absorbed individual loses sensitivity to others. His feelings become deficient for anyone outside of himself. Flouting conventional values as beneath him, the self-absorbed person makes his own rules and lets others be damned. Self-image is based on fantasy and exaggeration, to the point where the boundary between truth and lies is blurred. Rationalization runs rampant.

The rule breaker. In balance, this person is an iconoclast who does not follow the group. She is a shrewd operator, able to work around the system to accomplish worthwhile goals. Unbalanced, she lacks sensitivity to society at large. The serotonin-deficient individual can become overly impulsive and shortsighted, proceeding rashly without considering consequences.

It's important to remember that nobody is happy and stress-free all of the time, and we each have our share of emotional problems. However, if we don't address our negative issues, a bigger problem can emerge: in the face of a continued deficit of a vital brain chemical, a quirk that otherwise could easily be dismissed may turn into a full-blown psychiatric condition. Any serious condition, whether it be physical or psychological, begins as a minor one, and if you or someone close to you recognizes early signs of a personality imbalance, you can intervene by using one of the neurotransmitter-specific programs outlined in this book. This topic will be more thoroughly covered in Chapter 11.

NATURAL BRAIN FUNCTIONS

ATTENTION

A physiological function of the brain concerns your abilities to learn and remember. Attention deficits are generally thought to be associated mostly with children, but recent developments have led researchers to recognize that attention problems not only continue into the adult years for affected children but also reveal themselves in more of us as we age. Attention decreases can also be an early sign of Alzheimer's disease.

If you have been forgetting things lately, keep shifting from one activity to another, seem especially accident-prone, can't think clearly, suddenly start to feel either hyper or apathetic, or are finding it difficult to get along with family, friends, and colleagues, you may have an attention problem. These symptoms can be very disruptive, but researchers have found that problems of attention in adults are treatable. The solution can be found once again in one of the four neurotransmitters, a topic covered thoroughly in Chapter 10.

ATTENTION DEFICIT SYMPTOMS AND THEIR CAUSES

SYMPTOM	BIOCHEMICAL CAUSE
Inconsistent attention	Insufficient dopamine
Misplacing items, carelessness	Insufficient acetylcholine
Lack of attention, impulsive actions	Insufficient GABA
Inability to grasp concepts quickly	Insufficient serotonin

MEMORY

Lapses in memory are not an inevitable consequence of aging. They are a concrete indication of brain chemical deficiencies, and they can be reversed. While the primary neurotransmitter responsible for memory function is acetylcholine, each of the other three plays a role. If you experience any problems with memory, don't ignore them: once again, they are early warning signs of an underlying chemical deficiency. This topic will be more thoroughly covered in Chapter 11, but you should be aware of the four distinct types of memory, each ruled by one of the major neurotransmitters.

Working memory involves the ability to absorb information or stimuli and retain it for ongoing processing. It involves bringing together old and current data, and if the brain is overloaded with the latter, it will dump older memories. Working memory is affected by the frontal lobes and the biochemical dopamine.

Immediate memory, which lasts up to thirty seconds before the thought is transferred to long-term memory, consists of auditory and visual memory and is an indication of one's learning capabilities and basic alertness. Immediate memory is governed by the parietal lobe and the biochemical acetylcholine.

Verbal memory is necessary to produce and understand sound, words, sentences, and stories. Verbal memory is controlled by the temporal lobes and the biochemical GABA.

Visual memory involves the ability to absorb and retain information such as faces, colors, shapes, designs, surroundings, pictures, and symbols. People who can drive to a location after being there only once demonstrate excellent visual memory. Visual memory is assisted by the occipital lobes and the biochemical serotonin.

RETHINKING TOTAL HEALTH TREATMENT

The ultimate medical definition of life is brain electrical activity—if doctors cannot find signs of the brain working at a sufficient level, they sign a death certificate. Anatomically, the brain's structure is identical right before and immediately after death. Physiologically, it's quite a different story: after death all electrical activity ceases. Monitoring this electrical activity is how I assess health and determine what should be done to treat conditions and restore each patient's edge.

Being aware of brain-based symptoms that are related to specific anatomic functional areas—and the biochemicals related to them— enables us to take charge of our own health. Addressing the four key brain biochemicals and their electrical signals gets to the root of illness and is the path to total health.

Now that you understand the importance of the primary neurotransmitters, when mild symptoms first appear you can use this book to guide yourself toward readily available medications and natural therapies to recharge your brain. Appreciating the critical importance of the brain is the first step toward achieving a more abundant life.

2

ARE YOU LOSING YOUR EDGE?

LIVING AT YOUR peak—when every day is a good day at work, when enjoyment comes easily, and when you feel strong and healthy—can be directly traced to a balanced brain. This occurs when all four of your primary biochemicals (dopamine, acetylcholine, GABA, and serotonin) are transmitting properly and in the right proportions, your four electrical functions are working at optimal levels, the power supply is strong, brain speed is fast, rhythm is constant, and your brain is in sync. At this point, you are experiencing the Edge Effect.

However, if you are feeling ill and have physical complaints, you know intuitively that something is wrong. You might be experiencing symptoms that are not quite physical—they may be related to the mind and an overall feeling that you're not yourself. Regardless of the symptoms, the solution is to go to the source: your brain chemistry. If your brain chemistry is unbalanced, your body will be unbalanced. The moment you realize that something is off, you have already begun to lose your edge.

WHY WE HAVE UNBALANCED BRAINS

Some of us have always been off the edge to varying degrees. I call this being born edgy. Depending on which neurotransmitter is deficient, even a child as young as two or three years old will exhibit symptoms or a personality type that clearly define her as someone with poor health. A low-dopamine child might exhibit symptoms of ADD. A low-acetylcholine child may have learning disorders. A low-GABA child could have impulsive or violent tendencies, and a low-serotonin child might be moody or depressed.

Even those of us lucky enough to have experienced good health know that it is not possible for any of us to remain perfectly fit forever. Most of us will begin to lose our edge by the time we turn forty. We all have minor biochemical deficiencies that we have learned to live with. As we age, our bodies produce fewer of the hormones that regulate neurotransmitter production, throwing off a balance so delicate it can easily be upset simply by changing the output of one hormone. Imbalances are also affected by the day-to-day stresses of life and by the choices we make regarding what we eat. Over time, our brain will not be able to compensate for these consistent, seemingly minor assaults, and we develop what I refer to as a sprained brain.

While the body has remarkable capacities to heal itself, there are limits to what it can do on its own. For example, a minor cut on your finger will regenerate new skin within a week, but a bullet wound to the chest will require surgical intervention. Sprained brains work in the same manner. Insignificant injuries, such as the occasional down moment we've all experienced, usually reverse on their own with the help of a good night's sleep. More serious sprains, such as chronic pain or depression, must be accurately assessed and treated.

Between the two extremes are moderate imbalances. These are the ones to be most wary of, because if they are not addressed, what may seem like a small problem today might progress to something far worse in the future. This is like driving your car when you know that one tire is not properly balanced. The tire's tread will wear unevenly, and the slight effect that this has on the car's ride might not be noticeable at first. But uneven tread on one tire will lead to uneven tread wear on the other tires, with a subsequent effect on alignment. The car will then be harder to steer, and the brakes will wear out faster. Ignored, what would normally be just a simple matter of adjusting the wheel balance can lead to major expenses for new tires, brakes, shocks, and steering alignment.

The same is true for you. If you notice that you are losing your edge, you are probably experiencing deficiencies in your biochemistry. These deficiencies will eventually have a significant impact on how you feel. What you might have thought was a temporary symptom or a bad mood is actually a brain chemical reaction with far more serious implications. However, you can regain your edge by mastering your brain chemistry and putting yourself on the path back to health.

For example, a high-powered attorney might normally be insensitive to the feelings of others and uninterested in non-business-related diversions. A dopamine-driven person is perfectly willing to live like this: he might not even realize his behavior is out of the ordinary. Though he might relegate his health concerns to the back burner, once he develops high blood pressure he'll likely be sufficiently scared to seek medical attention. If he doesn't, at some point he won't be able to make the complicated strategic decisions that define him—or worse. If he had recognized that the changes in his thinking style were really a sign that he was slipping off the edge, and if he had acted on that knowledge, he could have prevented his new significant problem.

THE EDGE CHECKLIST

Are you experiencing any of the following major physical illnesses? While these all require immediate medical attention, they are also signs that you have lost your edge:

Anemia	Epstein-Barr syndrome	Nonconvulsive epilepsy
Arthritis		
Back pain	Glaucoma	Obesity
Cholesterol elevation	Head injury	Osteoporosis
Chronic pain	Hearing loss	Seizures
Cognitive thinking difficulty	Hypertension	Sexual dysfunction
	Kidney problems	Stroke
Concussion	Liver tumors	Vertigo
Delusions	Lyme disease	Viral infections
Depression	Memory loss	
Diabetes	Multiple sclerosis	

More moderate conditions, which we all have experienced and continue to endure, are probably more important to recognize. These are issues that you might have felt are too minor to require treatment or, worse, that you think are self-induced and will go away on their own.

In truth, these complaints can likely be traced once again to your biochemicals. So stop blaming yourself for what you might think of as "personality flaws." These conditions listed on the next page are important signals that you may be losing your edge:

Abnormal involuntary movements

Absentmindedness

Accident-proneness

An experience of feeling automated or as if in a dream

An experience that something is unfamiliar about familiar places or events

Anger management problems

Blurred vision

Constipation

Delays in processing information

Difficulty achieving orgasm

Digestive complaints

Distractedness

Dizziness or giddiness

Drug or alcohol addiction

Feeling detached, as if one is an outside observer of one's mental processes or body

Frequently interrupting others

Impotence

Increased impulsiveness

Lack of coordination

Low sex drive

Mood swings

Out-of-body experiences

Panic attacks

Perfectionism

Phobias, fears

Reactive confusion

Short temper

Shuffling gait

Shyness

Smell hallucinations

Spatial perception difficulties

Sweating

Taste hallucinations

Thought confusions

BENDING ONE'S CHEMISTRY THE WRONG WAY

You might have been living with these conditions or others for some time, and have been compensating for them indirectly. When we start to lose our edge, many of us unknowingly take treatment into our own hands. Some of us will seek medical attention for a particular ailment and treat it, which will work initially, until a new symptom pops up. Others might try to boost their energy by changing what they consume—for example, drinking coffee, smoking cigarettes, or eating lots of sweets just to stay alert—in a form of self-medication. Another group will try to stabilize their environment by becoming cautious, and take themselves outside of society if they are afraid of how they might function around others. Then there are those who just don't care. When they start losing the edge, they binge or eat unhealthy foods, drink excessive quantities of alcohol, and find jobs that require minimal cognitive ability because they can't rely on their intellectual processing.

The most dramatic example of self-medication is the abuse of drugs. Cocaine, for one, provides a short-term burst of energy, mimicking the effect of dopamine. But as the brain becomes accustomed to cocaine's high, it compensates by reducing its own dopamine production. This, in turn, increases the body's demand for dopamine, which then can only be supplied by increased amounts of cocaine. The result is a vicious circle in which the addict continually needs higher doses of cocaine, and which ends when the brain totally burns itself out of dopamine. Hallucinogenic mushrooms work similarly on acetyl-choline, marijuana and quaaludes on GABA, and the club drug Ecstasy on serotonin. All of these addictive cycles end up as major physical and psychiatric disorders unless the drug abuser can find a way to stop.

You don't have to be a drug addict to upset the balance of your brain chemistry. Millions of people do themselves harm through legal and socially accepted means. You might drink gallons of coffee and eat lots of sugar to increase your energy—a dopamine high. Perhaps you get an acetyl-choline boost in the form of a regular nicotine fix to help yourself think clearly, or you binge on carbohydrates, a GABA tranquilizer, to feel better. Maybe you consume alcohol, a serotonin enhancer, a little too often so that you can shut down and get to sleep. While self-medicating through diet might seem to work in the short term, it only provides the illusion of solving the problem, and over time it can negatively affect your health. The damage from these everyday habits can be as serious as that from drug addiction—it will just take a little longer to show up.

BENDING ONE'S CHEMISTRY THE RIGHT WAY

Instead of these quick fixes, there are effective treatments that can reverse the symptoms of a sprained brain. When biochemicals are adjusted to compensate for either an excess or a deficiency, you will have effectively bent your brain back in the other direction. For the most part, the place to begin is by addressing deficiencies. In some cases, such as a dopamine type subject to mania (due to too much dopamine), simply boosting calming GABA and serotonin may not be sufficient, so we'd need to use beta-blockers to stop the overproduced dopamine from being taken up by the cells. By adjusting brain chemistry, instead of treating only the immediate symptoms, you will have regained your edge, benefiting your whole mind and body.

By balancing your brain you can also improve your brain's cognitive functions, including your memory and attention. For example, with today's "smart drugs" and biochemical enhancers, you can lower your brain age and improve age-related memory loss. Make no mistake: if you put in the proper effort, you can rebuild your health and reverse brain aging. What's more, by balancing it all, you will achieve the Edge Effect for total brain and body health.

Regaining our edge can also lead to the ability to modify our personalities. We can learn to bolster our behavioral weaknesses, which are often the opposites of our temperament. For example, the organized individual can become more spontaneous; the thinker can increase his empathy; the introvert can learn to build multiple relationships; and intuitives can become more logical.

You might be surprised to find how simple and straightforward the balanced-brain approach is. At the first sign of health problems, you can choose from several therapies to address your sprained brain and restore it to its optimal working order. I guarantee that if you make even a few of the changes I suggest in the pages that follow, you will be closer to achieving total health, because it all begins with the brain.

DETECTING THE UNBALANCED BRAIN

Your dominant biochemical controls your temperament, or what I call your nature. Your nature encompasses all of the physical, mental, and emotional aspects of your health. If a patient comes to me with a physical problem such as chronic headaches, I can predict that she also has other issues, whether or not she's aware of them. Perhaps this patient has had subtle, low-grade depression, chronic anxiety, or an overall sense of malaise. Another patient might come to see me for asthma treatment, but when I probe further, it turns out he also has a memory deficit. These disorders are linked because they are nature-related illnesses.

When I can help patients balance their dominant biochemical, their health improves on every front. Nine times out of ten, mental or emotional aspects of the nature's deficiency are also resolved. With this book as your guide, you can evaluate and maintain your day-to-day health by identifying your dominant nature and determining whether you have a deficiency associated with it.

Sylvia came to see me at the age of twenty-eight with asthma so severe that she was frequently spending time in emergency rooms fighting for breath. Inhalers were not doing the job, and other medications seemingly had no effect. No matter what Sylvia took, the asthma worsened. Sylvia was a third-grade teacher, and her mounting sick days were becoming a real problem.

There was no doubt that Sylvia had a respiratory disorder. There was also no doubt that something else was going on, something that could be better understood if we identified Sylvia's dominant nature. It seemed to me that her brain chemical deficiency was causing her whole body to spasm. Because her lungs were her weak area, they were tightening up and producing asthmatic symptoms. But pulmonary drugs were not working for her because the source of her problem was not her lungs. I was able to identify her dominant GABA nature, and revealed a severe GABA deficiency that was the common denominator for all of her symptoms. Using GABA treatments, I properly addressed her biochemical nature and cured Sylvia in two weeks. Today she is feeling great and hasn't taken a sick day in more than a year.

HEALTHY CHOICES FOR
A BALANCED BRAIN

In the right environment and under the right supervision, you can control, modify, or enhance your brain chemistry just as Sylvia did. Using my unique approach, you will be able to work with your doctor to design an individual treatment program based on one or a combination of the seven types of therapies: medications, hormones, vitamins and supplements, diet, lifestyle, environment, and technology. The following is a broad introduction to these treatments. These positive alterations to your nature will alleviate symptoms, increase your energy, boost your immune system, keep you on an even keel, and help you achieve total health by restoring your edge.

MEDICATIONS

Medications are Western science's single greatest achievement, and they definitely have their place in restoring brain chemistry. Pharmaceuticals can impact chemical reactions at any stage to achieve a specific effect.

For example, some medications are designed to increase neurotransmitter production, while others reduce it. Some medications prevent or enhance neurotransmitter storage, while others prevent or enhance its transmission. Pharmaceuticals also work by mimicking the properties and metabolism of the various neurotransmitters. Or the metabolism of biochemicals can be transformed to stop the way the body uses up a neurotransmitter. For example, carbidopa-levodopa (Sinemet), a medication commonly prescribed for Parkinson's disease, enhances production of dopamine and prevents its breakdown in the body. Fluoxetine (Prozac), on the other hand, enhances serotonin transmission and preserves it, while diazepam (Valium) mimics the effects of additional GABA.

Whatever their ultimate goal, prescription drugs have the fastest and most powerful impact on a biochemical imbalance. Many of my patients need prescription drugs to get them back on track and help them regain their edge. However, my goal is always to use prescription drugs carefully and for as short a time as possible. Once a prescribed medication has accomplished the initial restoration of chemical balance, other, gentler alternatives can sustain it. These can be vitamin and mineral supplements or changes to your diet, lifestyle, and environment.

Prescription medications can have serious side effects, such as addiction and hypertension. The need to be seen regularly by a physician to monitor those potential side effects is why many prescriptions have limited—or no—refills. Never take medications given to you by even the most well-intentioned friend or loved one. Instead, prescriptions should always be taken under the supervision of a medical doctor. Make it a practice to throw away leftover medications, and do not self-prescribe what you think is best for a particular illness. While I will show you how certain medications can be used for other functions than those initially prescribed, never take any prescription medication without consulting with your doctor first.

HORMONES

Ninety percent of all hormones are produced in or regulated by the brain. They are the brain's messengers, which are sent to all other parts of the body to control the specific functions of cells and organs. Hormone replacement therapy can effectively alter brain chemical processes, although not as quickly as prescription medications.

As we age, our hormone-producing organs and glands begin to wear out. Their output drops, and the corresponding parts of the body begin to break down. The brain has to work harder as it tries to compensate for diminished body functions. This places a strain on the system, which then develops symptoms that lead us to seek treatment. If the decline in hormones is not treated, or if it is treated improperly, these biochemicals will be reduced further, resulting in more serious conditions.

Hormonal impact on brain function is indisputable. Research studies and clinical applications with thousands of patients have demonstrated the positive effect that hormones can have on neurotransmitter deficiency conditions, such as diminished concentration, memory loss, nicotine cravings, and insomnia, among others.

I prescribe hormone replacement therapies for my patients to address conditions that involve hormone deficiencies, ranging from menopause and andropause (the male equivalent of female hormonal changes) to sexual dysfunction, osteoporosis, mood disorders, fatigue, obesity, and cognitive deficiencies. However, the key component of my therapies is the use of natural, bioidentical hormones. These hormones are made from natural sources, such as plants, and work by precisely duplicating the body's original hormones.

The bonding of a hormone to its receptor is determined by the shape of the hormone molecule, like a key fits in a lock. Synthetic hormone molecules (not found in nature) and molecules from different species (Premarin, for example, is estrogen taken from female horses) differ in their molecular configuration from endogenous (made in the body) hormones, so they will also differ in their activity at the receptor level. This means they will not provide the same total activity as the hormones they are intended to replace, and that they will provoke side effects not found with the human hormone. Pharmaceutical companies, however, prefer synthetic hormones. Synthetic hormones can be patented, whereas natural, bioidentical hormones cannot.

For years I have rebuked the medical establishment for its widespread use of substances that have deleterious effects, and like the early vitamin pioneers, I've finally been vindicated. Studies of women given synthetic estrogen now show a 100 percent increase in risk of blood clots (a primary cause of stroke), a 40 percent increase in heart attacks, and a 26 percent increase in breast cancer, compared to women in a control group who were given a placebo. Women who've been using natural, bioidentical estrogen have not suffered these harmful effects.

As with pharmaceuticals, hormones can be abused. Because hormones directly affect internal chemistry, they should be used judiciously and under the direction of a doctor.

DIET

You might think that the foods you eat go directly to your stomach (or your thighs), but everything we put into our mouth first affects our brain. For example, think about how sleepy you feel after eating a big plate of pasta at lunchtime, or how you crave carbohydrates when you are under stress. It's common sense, then, to learn to eat to your advantage by understanding the specific impacts different foods have on our natures.

A great example of food chemistry is coffee. Heading out for a long drive? A little coffee is a good choice. But if you drink coffee all day long, you'll end up nervous, irritable, and unable to sleep. You'll spike your dopamine and strain both your GABA and serotonin as they try to calm you down.

Amino Acids: Protein-Building Neurotransmitters

Of the four essential nutrient groups, the most fundamental to brain chemistry is protein and its building blocks, amino acids. Amino acids are the precursors to neurotransmitters, and the production of these biochemicals can be directly affected by amino acids in your diet. The list on the next page shows which amino acids are necessary to increase the production of a specific neurotransmitter.

However, the chemical composition of food is complex. Food sources that support specific natures still contain nutrients that affect

NEUROTRANSMITTER	AMINO ACID NEEDED TO PRODUCE IT
Dopamine	Tyrosine
Acetylcholine	Phosphatidylserine, Acetyl-L-carnitine
GABA	Glutamine
Serotonin	Tryptophan

the others. For example, turkey, which is high in tryptophan—the primary building block for serotonin—also contains the amino acid that is needed to produce dopamine. Eggs, which provide a terrific boost for acetylcholine, have a glutamine component that helps support GABA. This is one of the reasons foods take longer to have their effect, and often need to work in conjunction with other modifications—whether they be prescription drugs, hormones, food supplements, or environmental changes.

Learning to make better dietary choices based on your nature can help you maintain better, balanced health, but you won't see changes in a matter of minutes, as you do with medication, or in a matter of days, as is the case with hormones. Altering your nature through diet requires weeks. But diet is far gentler on your body, supports your body's natural mechanisms for neurotransmitter production, and results in a stable, long-term balance.

Does a nature-based diet mean you can't have any fun? Do you have to give up chocolate, empty carbohydrates, sweets, or alcohol depending on your type? Definitely not. It does mean that you may have to indulge in some of these choices less frequently. Far more important, once you identify a deficiency in one or more biochemicals, you need to consume the best foods for those specific neurotransmitters. If you choose the nutrients that support health now, you can help yourself avoid more serious ailments later. More important, you can reach the full Edge Effect by combining nature-specific diets. For example, combine the recommendations for dopamine and acetylcholine for maximum brain power, or combine the GABA and serotonin diets for maximum calming effects.

Vitamins and Supplements

Vitamins and other nutrients are found in a variety of healthy food sources. Yet our less-than-perfect daily lives often interfere with the ability to receive all the nutrients we desperately need. Being constantly on the go, traveling, commuting, and shuttling our children around, sometimes we're just too busy to restock our cupboards or fuss with meal preparation.

Whenever you miss nutritious meals, you're not only depleting your nature but also starving your brain. It can take just a few days to see some of the effects: irritability, loss of concentration, disturbed sleep. But help is readily available. Supplements not only enhance the effectiveness of even a well-balanced diet but also can serve as a temporary substitute when a proper diet regimen is not observed.

Like medications, hormones, and diet, vitamins and other supplements operate on the biochemical level: they initiate reactions, provide energy, help to break down substances, or aid in restoring a depleted element. It is no surprise that they can alter the four biochemical natures. Chromium, rhodiola, and thiamine help to build dopamine, for example; manganese, lipoic acid, and huperzine-A address acetylcholine; inositol, B vitamins, and branched-chain amino acids are GABA-related; and vitamin B_6, St. John's wort, and fish oils are used for serotonin-based therapies.

The diets and supplement programs listed in this book are designed to work together. Specifically, the diets promote the absorption of the supplements. Therefore, for best results, use both these programs together.

LIFESTYLE

The term *lifestyle* covers a broad spectrum of behaviors. When we talk about changing our lifestyles, we usually are referring to slowing down our hectic schedules or becoming more physically active. These changes are a simple way to restore and maintain a balanced nature. They provide the means for the brain to replenish itself during the day as well as at night.

No doubt the most pervasive lifestyle issue is stress. Every job has a certain amount of stress associated with it, including unrealistic deadlines, undercompensation, deadly monotony, or friction with supervisors or coworkers. But stress has its positive side. Moderate amounts of stress cause the body to produce dopamine, which gives us the energy to perform, to get things done without procrastinating, to plan, to work hard, and to achieve.

You don't have to change your life radically in order to find activities that will reduce stress. A one-hour power nap, for example, is perfect for giving the brain a chance to restore its neurotransmitters naturally. And there's no lack of evidence about the efficacy of regular physical exertion in improving health. However, if you want to restore a deficient neurotransmitter, the exercise you pick is key. Weight-bearing exercise builds dopamine, while more aerobic activity such as running or swimming supports the other three natures.

Like diet, changes in lifestyle take time to affect brain chemistry, but I guarantee that you will see results. A game of chess increases dopamine; writing a letter replenishes some acetylcholine; a nature walk heightens GABA; sculpting can support your serotonin. Yet even play can have a negative effect if carried to extremes. If you are constantly seeking thrills and mind-expanding experiences—hang gliding, roller-coaster riding, skydiving—you are actually burning out your body's ability to produce acetylcholine the same way LSD would. Once again the answer is maintaining balance, and taking everything, even leisure time, in moderation.

Meditation, chanting, and prayer—important aspects of spirituality—have calming effects that allow the brain to slow down and resynchronize. However, belief in a supreme being, an afterlife, or reincarnation isn't a prerequisite for reaping the rewards of spiritual practice. Like spirituality, nurturing relationships allow your brain to relax. Relationships fraught with stress and antagonism eventually deplete your supply of all four neurotransmitters. A pattern of healthy, rewarding relationships—with associates, friends, or loved ones—can have lifelong advantages.

ENVIRONMENT

The word *environment* has come to mean many things to many people. When I use the word, some of my patients think I'm talking about lead poisoning, PCBs, toxic metals in our water, acid rain, global warming, nuclear waste, ozone depletion, and pesticides. Others assume I'm referring to problems associated with cell phones and microwave ovens. Sadly, all of these environmental dangers are real. Their effects can be subtle, but over time they can and will damage your mind and body.

Thirty years ago, when I first began researching the effects of lead in people who worked in battery factories, very few of my peers could believe the disturbing data. Since then, numerous studies have proven beyond a doubt that lead decreases GABA, cadmium in cigarette smoke decreases dopamine, exposure to the light from fluorescent bulbs and to the aluminum in cookware or drinking water decreases acetylcholine, and pesticides decrease serotonin. Less well documented are the effects of the media's environmental assaults—violent films, pornography, loud music, and foul language. I believe that exposure to such personal upsets depresses production of GABA, acetylcholine, and serotonin.

Though you might not see a difference overnight, you will be amazed at how significantly your overall health changes once you remove harmful environmental influences from your daily life, especially those that affect your nature directly. By changing your environment, you're enhancing the best properties of the Edge Effect, often with little effort.

TECHNOLOGICAL BREAKTHROUGHS

A more direct intervention against environmental hazards and other biochemical damage involves the use of technology in an innovative and beneficial way, through devices that employ electrical or magnetic stimulation. I've had good results with my patients when I have prescribed the following treatments. All require a prescription or an office visit and are available through your doctor or pharmacist. Discuss their use with your doctor before you proceed with any of them.

Transcutaneous electrical nerve stimulation (TENS) units have long been used to relieve pain and promote localized healing. They are small—about the size of a cell phone—and they apply tiny amounts of electricity via electrodes that are affixed to specific areas of the body. TENS units stimulate the release of endorphins, which are the body's own pain medication. The electrical stimulation of muscles through these units induces mild contractions that help to restore strength to atrophied muscles.

The *cranial electrical stimulator (CES)* is similar in size and electrical function to TENS units. With the CES, the electrodes are placed on the left wrist—site of the left vagal nerve, which connects directly to the midbrain—and on the forehead near the frontal lobes, which are the brain's pacemaker. The low voltage administered by the CES increases neurotransmitter levels—it's a catalyst for the amino acid conversions of glutamine into GABA and tryptophan into serotonin. The CES is FDA-approved for treatment of anxiety, depression, and insomnia—conditions directly related to GABA and serotonin deficiencies. Research also suggests that the CES device can be used as an antidote to damaging electromagnetic fields from microwaves, televisions, cell phones, and computers.

Transcranial magnetic stimulation (TCMS) units, a modification of the TENS units, have been developed for chronic pain and depression, both serotonin-deficient maladies. It makes perfect sense to me that the antidote for an electrical problem would be a brain balancer such as a TCMS unit. These handheld units utilize magnetism instead of direct electrical current to affect brain waves. Insulated coils generate magnetic fields that in turn generate electrical activity within specific brain lobes depending upon where the unit is applied. Studies have demonstrated that motor responses such as a twitching thumb can be induced by TCMS, memory and reaction time can be improved, and mood can be elevated. To date, they have shown early promise for stimulating the production of serotonin and GABA, which would help in treating depression, anxiety, and Alzheimer's disease.

THE NEXT STEP

The next step on your path to wellness is to identify your primary nature and learn to work with the biochemical that governs it. Understanding your dominant nature will help you identify potential illnesses you might develop, and guide you toward the best ways to prevent them. You will learn which medications, hormones, foods, and supplements can enhance your nature and bring you closer to the Edge Effect by boosting biochemical production.

Recognizing your dominant nature can also help you to understand, modify, and ultimately balance your personality. There comes a time when our natures do not serve us well: what was once a positive attribute can become a problem in a new context. For example, an extremely driven high-dopamine student will likely excel at school but might turn off people in the workplace with behavior that might be considered overbearing. Learning to balance your temperament with

the best characteristics of the three other natures is therefore as important as balancing your brain for overall health.

Obviously, there are more than four types of people. What makes
every one of us unique is that while we each have one dominant nature,
we also have differing amounts of the other three biochemicals. The
combinations are infinite. While your dominant nature will tell you
how to restore and maintain your health, you also may be deficient in
one of the other three biochemicals.

The relationship of brain biochemicals is similar to how the parts
of a car work together to get you where you need to go. Dopamine, like
gasoline, is a source of power; acetylcholine, like the accelerator, regulates speed; GABA, like the brakes, controls movement; and serotonin,
like the alternator, recharges the battery that starts the body's engine,
the brain. All four systems are necessary for a smooth ride. Each of us
functions in much the same way: you need to balance your nature with
the other three biochemicals, checking to see whether there is any other
deficiency that would cause your body to work at less than its full
potential.

Once you have defined your nature, you can begin the healing
process. You will be able to deal effectively with health issues that are the
result of imbalances in your brain biochemicals. You can quell that
craving for chocolate or address a more serious addiction to cigarettes
or alcohol. You will understand why you feel tired or why you are forgetting things more frequently. More important, you will learn what
you can do about these problems. You are taking control of your health
and happiness by regaining your edge.

3

WHICH NATURE ARE YOU?

YOUR NATURE DEFINES you. Specifically, your unique brain chemistry directly affects your memory, attention, personality, and physical health. The combination of the biochemicals dopamine, acetylcholine, GABA, and serotonin controls how you think, how you feel, and how you behave. Your dominant biochemical, which is the one your brain produces in the greatest quantity, governs the other three. Identifying your dominant biochemical, and in turn your dominant nature, is the key to self-discovery.

It is also important to know which biochemicals you are lacking, or not producing in sufficient quantities. These deficiencies are the direct causes of many medical problems. Knowing how to restore either your dominant nature or your secondary natures is the way to begin regaining your edge. By balancing them all, you will reach the full Edge Effect.

In order to identify both your dominant nature and possible biochemical deficiencies, I have developed a simple test that you can take in the privacy of your own home. My twenty-minute profile, which I call the Braverman Nature Assessment, identifies your dominant brain chemistry by both examining physical symptoms and evaluating the psychological dimensions of temperament, type, and personality. The assessment can also reveal the early stages of a brain biochemical deficiency, which will explain the subtle symptoms you experience when you don't feel quite right. The results of these tests then become the guide for all of your health-related issues.

Henry was suffering from chronic hypertension when he came in to see me. The powerful beta-blocker drugs that had been prescribed to lower his blood pressure were having serious side effects: depression, sexual dysfunction, fatigue, dizziness, and a weakened heart muscle. This, inevitably, had led to more prescription drugs: antidepressants, sildenafil (Viagra), and blood thinners. His blood pressure certainly came down, but was Henry in better health? He desperately wanted to get off the medication merry-go-round.

Conventional behavior tests identified Henry as a highly intelligent, driven person who was under heavy stress: the classic type-A personality. The treatment plan based on this information included lifestyle modification exercises and the continuation of the prescription drugs he was already taking. However, Henry's Nature Assessment revealed that although he did exhibit certain thinking and high-achieving characteristics associated with a dopamine nature, his true dominant nature was GABA. The solution to his condition was found in correcting a GABA imbalance, which we did through a combination of medication, diet, and supplements. Happily, Henry is no longer taking the majority of his medications, and he is much calmer now.

Hundreds of my patients have found themselves in a similar scenario. Often they are prescribed medications that do not match their nature. While the initial symptoms might go away at first, almost invariably new ones crop up because their basic biochemical imbalance has not been addressed. This is one of the most important reasons to identify your nature: so that you can take steps to address your biochemical imbalance and keep other related illnesses from occurring.

BEFORE YOU TAKE
THE NATURE ASSESSMENT

The Nature Assessment consists of two parts that contain series of true/false questions. The first part of the test determines your dominant nature. The second part will determine if you are experiencing any biochemical deficiencies.

Both tests should be completed in one sitting. Find a quiet place where you won't be distracted by music, nearby activities, or other people, and choose a time when you know that you will not be interrupted by phones, pagers, faxes, or e-mail. Lastly, check your physical state. Postpone taking the tests if you feel particularly out of sorts, or if you're not well rested and well fed.

The most important thing to remember is that there are no right answers to this assessment. You are born with your nature: there is no better or worse nature to have. We all have strengths and weaknesses. So don't overthink the questions, and don't answer as you might in a perfect world. If you want real insight into your overall health, answer truthfully.

Also, don't assume you know your nature before all the votes are counted. You will probably be surprised by the results; most people are. Try not to labor over the answers to a few of questions that you might not be sure about. The test is designed so that a few answers one way or another will not skew the result. Your first inclination, or gut reaction, always indicates the right way to answer the questions in these tests.

THE BRAVERMAN NATURE ASSESSMENT

PART 1: DETERMINING YOUR DOMINANT NATURE

Instructions: Answer each question by circling either T for true or F for false. At the end of each group, record only the total number of true statements in the space provided.

Answer the questions in terms of how you feel most of the time. For example, if you've had a bad night's sleep and feel tired today, answer the questions that pertain to your energy levels based on how you feel on a more average day.

1A
—

Memory and Attention
I find it easy to process my thoughts. T / F
I concentrate effectively. T / F
I am a deep thinker. T / F
I am a quick thinker. T / F
I become distracted because I do so many tasks at once. T / F
I enjoy intense debate. T / F
I have a good imagination. T / F
I tend to criticize and analyze my thoughts. T / F

Physical

I have a lot of energy most of the time. T / F

My blood pressure is often elevated. T / F

Sometimes in my life I have had episodes of extreme energy. T / F

I have insomnia. T / F

I find exercising invigorating. T / F

I don't ordinarily need coffee to jump-start me in
    the morning. T / F

My veins are visible and tend to look as though they might pop
    out of my skin. T / F

I tend to have a high body temperature. T / F

I eat my lunch while I'm working. T / F

I engage in sexual intercourse any chance I get. T / F

I have a temper. T / F

I eat only to reenergize my body. T / F

I love action movies. T / F

Exercising makes me feel powerful. T / F

Personality

I am a very domineering individual. T / F

I sometimes don't notice my feelings. T / F

I often have trouble listening to others because my own ideas domi-
    nate. T / F

I have been in many physical altercations. T / F

I tend to be future-oriented. T / F

I am sometimes speculative. T / F

Most people view me as thinking-oriented. T / F

I daydream and often fantasize. T / F

I like to read history and other nonfiction books. T / F

I admire ingenuity. T / F

I can be slow in identifying how people can cause trouble. T / F

I don't usually get tricked by people who say they need my help. T / F

Most people view me as innovative. T / F

People have thought I have had some strange ideas, but I can always
    explain the basis for them rationally. T / F

I am often agitated or irritated. T / F

Little things make me anxious or upset. T / F

I have fantasies of unlimited power. T / F

I love spending money. T / F

I dominate others in my relationships. T / F

I am very hard on myself. T / F

I react aggressively to criticism, often becoming defensive in front of others. T / F

Character

Some individuals view me as tough-minded. T / F

Most people view me as achievement-oriented. T / F

Some people say that I am irrational. T / F

I will do anything to reach a goal. T / F

I value a religious philosophy. T / F

Incompetence makes me angry. T / F

I have high standards for myself and for others. T / F

Total number of T responses: _____

2 A

Memory and Attention

My memory is very strong. T / F

I am an excellent listener. T / F

I am good at remembering stories. T / F

I usually do not forget a face. T / F

I am very creative. T / F

I have an excellent attention span and rarely miss a thing. T / F

I have many good hunches. T / F

I notice everything going on around me. T / F

I have a good imagination. T / F

Physical

I tend to have a slow pulse. T / F

My body has excellent tone. T / F

I have a great figure/build. T / F

I have low cholesterol. T / F

When I eat, I love to experience the aromas and the beauty of food. T / F

I love yoga and stretching my muscles. T / F

During sex I am very sensual. T / F

I have had an eating disorder at some point in my life. T / F

I have tried many alternative remedies. T / F

Personality

I am a perpetual romantic. T / F

I am in touch with my feelings. T / F

I tend to make decisions based on hunches. T / F

I like to speculate. T / F

Some people say I have my head in the clouds. T / F

I love reading fiction. T / F

I have a rich fantasy life. T / F

I am creative when solving people problems. T / F

I am very expressive; I like to talk about what's bothering me. T / F

I am buoyant. T / F

I believe that it is possible to have a mystical experience. T / F

I believe in being a soul mate. T / F

Sometimes the mystical can excite me. T / F

I tend to overreact to my body. T / F

I find it easy to change; I am not set in my ways. T / F

I am deeply in touch with my emotions. T / F

I tend to love someone one minute and hate him or her the next.
  T / F

I am flirtatious. T / F

I don't mind spending money if it benefits my relationships. T / F

I tend to fantasize when I'm having sex. T / F

My relationships tend to be filled with romance. T / F

I love watching romantic movies. T / F

I take risks in my love life. T / F

Character

I foresee a better future. T / F

I am inspired to help other people. T / F

I believe that all things are possible, particularly for those
  who are devoted. T / F

I am good at creating harmony between people. T / F

Charity and altruism come from the heart, and I have plenty of
  both. T / F

Others think me of as having vision. T / F
My thoughts on religion often change. T / F
I am an idealist, but not a perfectionist. T / F
I'm happy with someone who just treats me right. T / F

Total number of T responses: _____

3A

Memory and Attention
I have a stable attention span and can follow other people's logic.
   T / F
I enjoy reading people more than books. T / F
I retain most of what I hear. T / F
I can remember facts people tell me. T / F
I learn from my experiences. T / F
I am good at remembering names. T / F
I can focus very well on tasks and people's stories. T / F

Physical
I find it easy to relax. T / F
I am a calm person. T / F
I find it easy to fall asleep at night. T / F
I tend to have high physical endurance. T / F
I have low blood pressure. T / F
I do not have a family history of stroke. T / F
When it comes to sex, I am not very experimental. T / F
I have little muscle tension. T / F
Caffeine has little effect on me. T / F
I take my time eating my meals. T / F
I sleep well. T / F
I don't have many harmful food cravings such as sugar. T / F
Exercising is a regimented habit for me. T / F

Personality
I am not very adventurous. T / F
I do not have a temper. T / F
I have a lot of patience. T / F
I don't enjoy philosophy. T / F

I love watching sitcoms about families. T / F

I dislike movies about other worlds or universes. T / F

I am not a risk taker. T / F

I keep past experiences in mind before I make decisions. T / F

I am a realistic person. T / F

I believe in closure. T / F

I like facts and details. T / F

When I make a decision, it's permanent. T / F

I like to plan my day, week, month, etc. T / F

I collect things. T / F

I am a little sad. T / F

I'm afraid of confrontations and altercations. T / F

I save up a lot of money in the event of a crisis. T / F

I tend to create strong, lasting bonds with others. T / F

I am a stable pillar in people's lives. T / F

Character

I believe in the adage "Early to bed, early to rise." T / F

I believe in meeting deadlines. T / F

I try to please others the best I can. T / F

I am a perfectionist. T / F

I am good at maintaining long-lasting relationships. T / F

I pay attention to where my money goes. T / F

I believe that the world would be more peaceful if people would
improve their morals. T / F

I am very loyal and devoted to my loved ones. T / F

I have high ethical standards that I live by. T / F

I pay close attention to laws, principles, and policies. T / F

I believe in participating in service for the community. T / F

Total number of T responses: _____

4A

Memory and Attention

I can easily concentrate on manual-labor tasks. T / F

I have a good visual memory. T / F

I am very perceptive. T / F

I am an impulsive thinker. T / F

I live in the here and now. T / F

I tend to say, "Tell me the bottom line." T / F

I am a slow book learner, but I learn easily from experience. T / F

I need to experience something or work at it hands-on in order to understand it. T / F

Physical

I sleep too much. T / F

When it comes to sex, I am very experimental. T / F

I have low blood pressure. T / F

I am very action-oriented. T / F

I am very handy around the house. T / F

I am very active outdoors. T / F

I engage in daring activities such as skydiving and motorcycle riding. T / F

I can solve problems spontaneously. T / F

I rarely have carbohydrate cravings. T / F

I usually grab a quick meal on the run. T / F

I'm not very consistent with my exercise routine; I may exercise daily for three weeks and then skip it for a month. T / F

Personality

I live life in the immediate moment. T / F

I like to perform/entertain in public. T / F

I tend to gather facts in an unorganized manner. T / F

I am very flexible. T / F

I am a great negotiator. T / F

I often just like to "eat, drink, and be merry." T / F

I am dramatic. T / F

I am very artistic. T / F

I am a good craftsman. T / F

I'm a risk taker when it comes to sports. T / F

I believe in psychics. T / F

I can easily take advantage of others. T / F

I am cynical of others' philosophies. T / F

I like to have fun. T / F

My favorite types of movies are horror flicks. T / F

I am fascinated with weapons. T / F

I rarely stick to a plan or agenda. T / F

I have trouble remaining faithful. T / F

I am easily able to separate and move on when relationships with loved ones end. T / F

I don't pay much attention to how I spend my money. T / F

I have many frivolous relationships. T / F

Character

I always keep my options open in case something better comes up. T / F

I don't like working hard for long periods of time. T / F

I believe things should have a function and purpose. T / F

I am optimistic. T / F

I live in the moment. T / F

I pray only when I'm in need of spiritual support. T / F

I don't have particularly high morals and ethical values. T / F

I do what I want, when I want to. T / F

I don't care about being perfect; I just live my life. T / F

Savings are for suckers. T / F

Total number of T responses: _____

Results

1A. Total number of T responses: dopamine nature   ____

2A. Total number of T responses: acetylcholine nature   ____

3A. Total number of T responses: GABA nature   ____

4A. Total number of T responses: serotonin nature   ____

The category with the greatest number of true responses will identify your dominant nature. A classically dominant nature is typically a score of 35 and above in any one category, which suggests a less-than-balanced life.

Note: When any other nature is 10–15 points lower than the dominant one, the nature with the lower score is probably a lifelong relative deficiency and needs balance even in times of good health. For example, if your score is 40 dopamine, 33 acetylcholine, 25 GABA, and 17 serotonin, you likely have long-standing relative deficiencies in both GABA and serotonin.

PART 2: DEFINING YOUR DEFICIENCIES

Instructions: Answer each question by circling either T for true or F for false. At the end of each group, record only the total number of true statements in the space provided. The second assessment will determine if you are deficient in any of the four biochemicals, including the one that governs your nature. Many of the questions relate to symptoms you might be experiencing. Answer the questions in terms of how you feel right now; it doesn't matter how long you've been experiencing these symptoms, or even if they occurred today for the first time.

1B

Memory and Attention

I have trouble paying consistent attention and concentrating. T / F

I need caffeine to wake up. T / F

I cannot think quickly enough. T / F

I do not have a good attention span. T / F

I have trouble getting through a task even when it is interesting to me. T / F

I am slow in learning new ideas. T / F

Physical

I crave sugar. T / F

I have decreased libido. T / F

I sleep too much. T / F

I have a history of alcohol or addiction. T / F

I have recently felt worn out for no apparent reason. T / F

I sometimes experience total exhaustion without even exerting myself. T / F

I have always battled weight problems. T / F

I have little motivation for sexual experiences. T / F

I have trouble getting out of bed in the morning. T / F

I have had a craving for cocaine, amphetamines, or Ecstasy. T / F

Personality

I feel fine just following others. T / F

People seem to take advantage of me. T / F

I am feeling very down or depressed. T / F
People have told me I am too mellow. T / F
I have little urgency. T / F
I let people criticize me. T / F
I always look to others to lead me. T / F

Character
I have lost my reasoning skills. T / F
I can't make good decisions. T / F

Total number of T responses: _____

2B
—

Memory and Attention
I lack imagination. T / F
I have difficulty remembering names when I first
    meet people. T / F
I have noticed that my memory ability is decreasing. T / F
My significant other tells me I don't have romantic thoughts. T / F
I can't remember my friends' birthdays. T / F
I have lost some of my creativity. T / F

Physical
I have insomnia. T / F
I have lost muscle tone. T / F
I don't exercise anymore. T / F
I crave fatty foods. T / F
I have experimented with hallucinogens or other illicit drugs. T / F
I feel like my body is falling apart. T / F
I can't breathe easily. T / F

Personality
I don't feel joy very often. T / F
I feel despair. T / F
I protect myself from being hurt by others by never telling much
    about myself. T / F
I find it more comfortable to do things alone rather than in a
    large group. T / F
Other people get angrier about bothersome things than I do. T / F

I give in easily and tend to be submissive. T / F
I rarely feel passionate about anything. T / F
I like routine. T / F

Character

I don't care about anyone's stories but mine. T / F
I don't pay attention to people's feelings. T / F
I don't feel buoyant. T / F
I'm obsessed with my deficiencies. T / F

Total number of T responses: _____

3B

Memory and Attention

I find it difficult to concentrate because I'm nervous and
   jumpy. T / F
I can't remember phone numbers. T / F
I have trouble finding the right word. T / F
I have trouble remembering things when I am put on the spot. T / F
I know I am intelligent, but it is hard to show others. T / F
My ability to focus comes and goes. T / F
When I read, I find I have to go back over the same paragraph a
   few times to absorb the information. T / F
I am a quick thinker but can't always say what I mean. T / F

Physical

I feel shaky. T / F
I sometimes tremble. T / F
I have frequent backaches and/or headaches. T / F
I tend to have shortness of breath. T / F
I tend to have heart palpitations. T / F
I tend to have cold hands. T / F
I sometimes sweat too much. T / F
I am sometimes dizzy. T / F
I often have muscle tension. T / F
I tend to get butterflies in my stomach. T / F
I crave bitter foods. T / F
I am often nervous. T / F
I like yoga because it helps me to relax. T / F

I often feel fatigued even when I have had a good night's sleep. T / F

I overeat. T / F

Personality

I have mood swings. T / F

I enjoy doing many things at one time, but I find it difficult to decide what to do first. T / F

I tend to do things just because I think they'd be fun. T / F

When things are dull, I always try to introduce some excitement. T / F

I tend to be fickle, changing my mood and thoughts frequently. T / F

I tend to get overly excited about things. T / F

My impulses tend to get me into a lot of trouble. T / F

I tend to be theatrical and draw attention to myself. T / F

I speak my mind no matter what the reaction of others may be. T / F

I sometimes have fits of rage and then feel terribly guilty. T / F

I often tell lies to get out of trouble. T / F

I have always had less interest than the average person in sex. T / F

Character

I don't play by the rules anymore. T / F

I have lost many friends. T / F

I can't sustain romantic relationships. T / F

I consider the law arbitrary and without reason. T / F

I now consider rules that I used to follow ridiculous T / F

Total number of T responses: _____

4B

Memory and Attention

I am not very perceptive. T / F

I can't remember things that I have seen in the past. T / F

I have a slow reaction time. T / F

I have a poor sense of direction. T / F

Physical

I have night sweats. T / F

I have insomnia. T / F

I tend to sleep in many different positions in order to feel comfortable. T / F

I always awake early in the morning. T / F

I can't relax. T / F

I wake up at least two times per night. T / F

It is difficult for me to fall back asleep when I am awakened. T / F

I crave salt. T / F

I have less energy to exercise. T / F

I am sad. T / F

Personality

I have chronic anxiety. T / F

I am easily irritated. T / F

I have thoughts of self-destruction. T / F

I have had suicidal thoughts in my life. T / F

I tend to dwell on ideas too much. T / F

I am sometimes so structured that I become inflexible. T / F

My imagination takes over. T / F

Fear grips me. T / F

Character

I can't stop thinking about the meaning of life. T / F

I no longer want to take risks. T / F

The lack of meaning in my life is painful to me. T / F

Total number of T responses: _____

Results

1B. Total number of T responses: dopamine deficiency _____

2B. Total number of T responses: acetylcholine deficiency _____

3B. Total number of T responses: GABA deficiency _____

4B. Total number of T responses: serotonin deficiency _____

Circle the highest number. This is your most deficient nature, the one that is most likely to lead to illness. Your deficient nature can be the same as or different from your dominant nature. In fact, you'll most likely recognize deficits in your dominant nature sooner than you would in other aspects of your biochemistry, simply because you are used to behaving and feeling a specific way. You burn out your edge just by being yourself. For example, dopamine natures can push themselves too hard at work. Serotonin natures are known to overindulge, especially with alcohol, which would also lead to a biochemical imbalance. When GABA natures don't get enough sleep, they create problems for themselves. Overworking all of the other biochemicals will burn out your acetylcholine. The next four chapters outline treatment modalities for rebalancing any nature deficiency you might have. Balance your most deficient nature first. Then balance the other three to reach the Ultimate Edge Effect.

Any category with up to 5 true statements is considered a minor deficiency. Any category with between 6 and 15 true statements is considered a moderate deficiency. If you have more than 15 true statements in any one category, this indicates a major deficiency; I recommend that you get your doctor involved as soon as possible.

The assessment test will bring out two kinds of deficiencies. The first part of the test points up deficiencies that are the natural result of having one neurotransmitter as dominant. These deficiencies show up over time. The second part of the test uncovers deficiencies that may require more immediate attention.

Minor deficits are the early warning signs of health problems. If ignored, they will eventually lead to more serious deficiencies, ultimately affecting your dominant nature, even if they occurred in another nature. If you fall into the moderate deficit range, you probably have already sought medical treatment for any number of ailments related to that deficiency. Minor and moderate deficits can be treated without medications and usually respond to a combination of natural/nutritional, hormonal, and lifestyle changes.

Major deficits warrant medical treatment and should be addressed immediately. Deficits are treated as diseases—for example, Parkinson's disease, severe mood disorders, high blood pressure, memory loss, seizure disorders, depression, learning disabilities, attention deficit disorder, migraines, sleep disorders, irritable bowel syndrome, manic depression, and anxiety, among others. These conditions most likely require medications; nutritional, hormonal, and lifestyle changes are usually not enough to address them. If you experience any of these symptoms or illnesses, it is important to consult your doctor and get immediate treatment.

FREQUENTLY ASKED QUESTIONS

By now you may have many questions about your nature. Here are some answers to the questions I am most frequently asked:

Q. How can I be sure I've identified my dominant nature?

A. The Braverman Nature Assessment is based on tests related to brain temperaments and their deficiencies that have been developed and refined over the past fifty years. The assessment incorporates knowledge gained from observation and experiment that has been widely published, reviewed by the most eminent brain scientists, and confirmed in clinical settings.

You may have noticed the repetitive nature of various questions; this is deliberate so that no one question skews the overall result.

Q. How does a true-false test reveal brain chemistry?

A. The assessment is the beginning of an internal conversation, which can be continued with your doctor if necessary. No test can reveal brain chemistry completely. Your answers to these questions reveal patterns of thought and behavior that are directly related to the neurotransmitters in the brain. For example, the neurotransmitter dopamine is an excitatory biochemical that, in ample supply, provides you with physical energy, mental energy, intense motivation, high sex drive, quick thinking/processing speed, and an ability to fight off cravings. If you lack all or some of these abilities and behaviors (as the questions in this test will reveal), then we have discovered that you most likely have a dopamine deficiency.

The research is overwhelming. Loners, depressed people, and chronically introverted individuals all have been found to have dopamine deficiencies. Individuals who use dopamine agents such as caffeine or even amphetamines are extroverting their brain and will behave in a way that's different from how their nature would express itself. With the help of these dopamine enhancers, they will exhibit behavior similar to an individual who has a dopamine dominance.

If you are intuitive, with very active cognitive thought processes and high learning capacities, these characteristics have been linked to acetylcholine dominance. Deficiencies of this nature can be associated with attention disorders, psychosis, and nicotine addiction.

Q. How does the assessment differ from other widely known psychological profile tests?

A. The psychiatric profession has done remarkable work devising tests that reveal personality traits based on one's state of mind. A person's nature is the combination of personality, memory, attention, and physical health. The Braverman Nature Assessment is the first instrument that tests all of these domains.

Q. What if I couldn't easily decide on an answer for a large percentage of the questions?

A. Believe it or not, that in itself says something about your nature! It might be totally consistent with your dominant nature, and good health. However, if you are having trouble answering these questions, get a good night's sleep and try to take the test again. If you still feel uncertain about your answers, then it is very likely that indecision is showing up in other parts of your professional or daily life. In that case, a checkup with your doctor is recommended so that underlying illness can be eliminated as a cause for your wavering. You might also want to review the dopamine nature section. A dopamine nature is able to make clear decisions, and by following the recommendations in that section, you might be able to improve your decision-making ability.

Q. Would medications or medical conditions influence my Nature Assessment?

A. Drugs such as antibiotics and most over-the-counter medications for ailments like the common cold have no effect on the results. If you are taking mind-altering medications such as antidepressants or tranquilizers, or certain hormones, the results might reflect a changed nature. This does not mean, however, that you should stop taking these prescribed medications, or that you should not take the Braverman Nature Assessment. The benefit of taking your assessment while on medication is that it can let you know if you are overmedicating yourself or if you are deficient in one of the four biochemicals. Are you really in balance using the medication? You might find out you have been taking the wrong medication or an incorrect dosage.

Q. Is it possible to have more than one dominant nature?

A. No. In some people, however, there are two natures that are both highly influential in overall health and well-being. Many people will have one score higher than the others; this score reflects your dominant nature. But some people will have identical scores for two or more natures. In that case, we determine their dominant nature in another way. The natural progression of activity in the brain wave is from the frontal lobe (dopamine) to the temporal lobe (GABA) to the parietal lobe (acetylcholine) to the occipital lobe (serotonin). The dominance patterns of the four natures, relative to each other, follow the same progression, with the exception of GABA. So if, say, your scores are identical for dopamine and acetylcholine, your dominant nature is dopamine, because dopamine comes first in the sequence. If you had identical scores for the GABA and serotonin natures, your dominant nature is serotonin.

Q. Once I've identified my dominant nature, how can I interpret all four scores of my Braverman Nature Test together?

A. The Braverman Nature Assessment is unique in that it can readily identify the biological reasons behind the physical problems you are experiencing now, as well as helping you balance your brain and body for the rest of your life. This information is determined by analyzing all four scores on the Nature Assessment.

Aside from your dominant nature, the next most important piece of information is held in your lowest score. This score identifies your weak side or, as I like to call it, your opposite nature. For example, if your test scores read 33 dopamine, 40 acetylcholine, 15 GABA, and 25 serotonin, you would be an acetylcholine nature with a GABA opposite nature. Remember, the natural progression of a brain wave is from the frontal lobe (dopamine) to the temporal lobe (GABA) to the parietal lobe (acetylcholine) to the occipital lobe (serotonin). The four natures follow the same progression, with the exception of GABA. If you had two identical lowest scores (e.g. 15 dopamine, 15 serotonin), the nature that appears first in the sequence would be considered your opposite nature. However, if you had identical low scores for GABA and serotonin, your opposite nature is serotonin.

While it is important to identify your dominant nature, you will not be able to reach the Ultimate Edge Effect unless you learn to balance all four natures. The first step then is to recognize and enhance your dominant nature through the nature-specific programs. Then, once you are well, you can begin to get your opposite nature into shape. Last, follow the programs for the two remaining natures. When all of your natures are balanced, you will reach the Ultimate Edge Effect and experience optimal health.

Q. What is the relationship between my dominant nature and my deficiencies?

A. Most people can identify a deficiency in their dominant nature before a deficiency in any other nature. This occurs when we feel less "like ourselves." However, compare your opposite nature in the Braverman Nature Assessment to your deficient nature in the second part of the test. In most cases, you will find that they are the same. This proves the brain's and body's desire to maintain balance. When this occurs your body is telling you to strive for the balance of where you were before. However, that balance should not be your entire goal. To get to the Ultimate Edge Effect, you can reach a state where you experience the full intensity, full enthusiasm, full organization, and full serenity of total balance. This can only be achieved by enhancing each corner of the edge, and working on all of your natures.

Q. Is there a connection between building successful relationships and identifying my dominant nature?

A. Yes! Your nature is an important facet in determining your biotemperament and personality, as well as identifying an ideal partner for your particular wants and desires. As the saying goes, opposites attract. You may find that your spouse or partner has the qualities found in your opposite nature. If this is so, you probably have a well-balanced relationship based on filling each other's weaknesses, and enhancing each other's strengths.

Conversely, the natures are paired by their correlation to the binary on/off switches of the brain. These pairs also make for dynamic relationships. For example, dopamine and acetylcholine are the binary "on" switches related to quickness and speed: intensity and enthusiasm in romance, love, and sex. An acetylcholine nature is fast, and usually expresses a high level of intensity of feeling, where romance dominates life. When dopamine is dominant, it serves cognitive efficiency. Together, they are a mark of high-voltage romantic loving. This coupling is what Hollywood romances strive for: the mark of the Western romantic mind and Western romantic thought. On the other hand, the "off" switches of GABA and serotonin often pair together. GABA natures have a calm sensibility, as well as the empathetic ability to give pain relief. When combined with serotonin where GABA is dominant, the coupling of the two maximizes the pain-free, easy-caring Eastern lifestyle. When serotonin is dominant, happiness, joy, and laughter in all its healing power are emphasized.

Stable relationships can also be found when you pair with the same nature. However, inevitably someone falls into a deficiency, and this type of relationship will suffer when the other can't adjust to the imbalance.

In all of these relationships, lifelong balance cannot be maintained by your choices of romantic pairings. Human nature drives us to try to change our partner instead of doing the work on ourselves when we recognize a problem. Therefore, the mark of a failing relationship is when people try to pull each other into their nature. Instead, you need to balance yourself by enhancing each of the four biochemical natures.

Q. At what age can you assess your dominant nature?

A. Many of the questions that constitute this test are not appropriate for children. I recommend first testing around the age of thirteen, when puberty most likely has begun. At that age the sexes diverge and our personality and temperament truly define our total selves. When testing younger patients, parents should be present and ensure that inappropriate questions are passed over. Skipping a small number of questions will not bias the result.

Q. What does it mean if I have multiple deficiencies?

A. Deficiencies in areas other than your dominant nature often show up as illness before a dominant nature deficiency reveals itself (which makes you feel like "you're not yourself"). Many health conditions present themselves as a series of multiple complex symptoms that can be traced to more than one nature. Treatment therefore must address multiple chemical imbalances. For example, memory problems associated with the acetylcholine nature are often accompanied by sleep abnormalities caused by a serotonin deficiency. If you are showing moderate or major deficiencies in multiple categories, make sure to review all of the respective sections to get a full picture of your current health.

Q. Can my dominant nature change over time? If so, how do I know?

A. Dominant natures do not change. They are established when you are born and become fully mature by the onset of puberty, around the age of thirteen. The health or balance of our dominant nature can change periodically, however. For example, you can have a dopamine-dominant nature and develop a dopamine deficiency. You would realize this problem if you scored high in both parts of the test within the same category (in this case, high scores in both 1A and 2A).

We are all a mixture of various natures. Generally speaking, we always have one dominant nature. However, there is no question that natures can vacillate: you might be stronger in one nature today and dominant in another when you feel more rested. Biochemical temperaments can also fluctuate due to illness. Sometimes people do not clearly know themselves, or have difficulty identifying symptoms that they are experiencing.

Q. Can I take the Braverman Nature Assessment again? If so, how long should I wait?

A. Although your dominant nature essentially does not change, you can alter it slightly based on how you take care of your body and mind. You can use Part 2 of the test as a way to determine your success in balancing your own brain chemistry.

Retake the Braverman Assessment whenever you feel markedly different for a week or more, make a major change to your vitamin or medication program, or experience a life-changing event such as the death of a loved one, a divorce, or a major illness. Always allow at least one month between assessments. It is not as important to define your dominant nature as it is to have the ability to balance your brain and use the strengths of all the natures to your benefit.

If your results show an even split among all natures (no one is dominant), then you are close to balancing your brain. If this is the case, then you are ready to augment your nature by boosting the biochemical you find most appealing to your temperament. For example, if you would like to be more outgoing, you can learn how to boost your dopamine; if you want to think more creatively, you can increase your acetylcholine levels.

Q. What role does genetics play in determining my dominant nature?

A. Genetics are key to your dominant nature. Individuals who exhibit dominance in a specific nature are predisposed to higher production and transmission of that specific neurotransmitter. You can also be predisposed to illnesses caused by the deficiencies in genes or in other natures. Our research shows that low dopamine, for example, is associated with obesity, addiction, alcoholism, antisocial behavior, and shyness.

Q. If I boost one neurotransmitter, isn't that going to create a new imbalance?

A. Every brain naturally functions at some level of imbalance. That is what makes each of us unique. The results from the Braverman Nature Test will therefore show some preference for one nature over another. You can also choose to augment a nature as needed: if you need to work late, you can rev up your dopamine; if you are going to an opera and need to sit still, you can rev up your acetylcholine and GABA. You are not creating an imbalance but enhancing a nature—and you are doing so on a temporary basis. This will not change the way your brain functions. You are simply increasing the output of a particular biochemical.

TOWARD BALANCE

You've now identified your dominant nature and discovered deficiencies you may have in the other natures. The rest of the book will show you how to optimize your dominant nature, reverse any deficiencies you might have, and keep the four neurotransmitters balanced for daily, lasting health.

Your dominant nature determines how you should be treated for any condition and how you can maintain your best health. By identifying this biochemical, you will be able to foresee possible medical conditions and take steps to prevent them. What's more, you will be able to boost your memory. Finally, you will better understand what drives your personality, and learn ways to modify its less-than-ideal aspects.

Part II of the book outlines four distinct programs for total health. Each of them represents one of the dominant natures and contains a diversified plan to address its specific needs. First, read the chapter about your dominant nature. Then read the chapter on the nature you are most deficient in. The combination of those two will be your personalized blueprint for optimal health. You can enhance this understanding by reading about the two remaining natures, especially if you have a specific ailment that is not covered in the first two natures. For example, if your energy levels are low, read the dopamine chapter. The acetylcholine chapter might solve your memory problems. If you are feeling anxious, read more about GABA. And if you need to figure out how to get a better night's sleep, check out the serotonin chapter.

PART II

RECOVERING

YOUR EDGE

4

THE POWERFUL
DOPAMINE NATURE

IF DOPAMINE IS most prevalent in your brain chemistry, you have a dopamine nature. Associated with high-voltage beta waves from your brain, dopamine affects the power of your body and mind. High-dopamine individuals like yourself are often powerful, reflexively fast, and quick-witted. When feeling well, people with dopamine natures have a very sharp edge.

In this chapter you will learn how to recognize the many aspects of your dopamine nature, and see how this biochemical affects all areas of your physical and mental health. More important, you will be able to recognize some of the specific symptoms you might be experiencing, and learn the correct way to fix a dopamine deficiency. By addressing this deficiency, you will be taking both a step toward better health and a leap toward attaining the Edge Effect.

THE DOPAMINE NATURE
PERSONALITY PROFILE

As a dopamine nature, you are among approximately 17 percent of the world's population. You thrive on energy. When your dopamine production is balanced, you are likely to be a strong-willed individual who knows exactly what you want and how to get it. You're fast on your feet and self-confident. You're highly rational, more comfortable with facts and figures than with feelings and emotions. You are able to assess yourself critically, yet you generally do not respond well to criticism or accept negative feedback from others.

You focus intently and persistently on the task at hand and take pride in achievement. Strategic thinking, masterminding, inventing, problem solving, envisioning, and pragmatism are exciting, and you function well under stress. These skills lend themselves to positions requiring complex knowledge and/or detailed planning. A majority of doctors, scientists, researchers, inventors, engineers, generals, and architects are likely to be dopamine-dominant. But this does not preclude other professions from dopamine natures: dopamine-dominant people can be found in every walk of life.

With a dopamine nature, you're most likely to be interested in activities related to knowledge and intellect. You might play chess, listen to books on tape, or do challenging crossword puzzles. You relish competition. You're tireless, perhaps hyperalert, and might require less sleep than your friends or family.

When it comes to physical activity, you find great satisfaction in anaerobic, weight-bearing exercises. You may also enjoy competitive individualized sports such as tennis, swimming, or skiing. If you follow professional sports, you might be as intrigued by the statistics of the sport as by the actual game being played.

Because rationality is your primary trait, you are more adept at establishing relationships than nurturing them. You're not overly sensitive, so you tend to miss the fact that others may believe their feelings are more powerful than reason. A successful marriage for a dopamine nature depends upon the loyalty and goodwill of the spouse. Relations with children could be distant and depend heavily on your ability to control the rest of the family.

The dopamine Edge Effect occurs when you've maximized your dopamine nature. These are the times when you experience total sensual enjoyment, you derive pleasure from everything you do, and your reactions are sharp. All of your senses are heightened: you relish sexual relations, your food tastes fantastic, and you feel powerful and admired among your friends and family.

TOO MUCH DOPAMINE

It is possible to have too much of a good thing. Dopamine natures who produce excessive amounts of this biochemical are at risk when their edge becomes too sharp. Producing too much dopamine makes you overly intense, driven, and impulsive. For example, while average dopamine types are intrigued by mental and physical stimulation, if they are over-producing this neurotransmitter, they may resort to violence as a way of creating controlled scenarios of excitement and power. Dopamine teens first learning to balance their edge might be driven to date rape, reckless driving, or shoplifting. At the extreme, criminals, especially repeat sexual offenders, are often high-dopamine natures with overactive libidos.

OUT OF BALANCE: DOPAMINE DEFICIENCY

If you scored high for dopamine in the second test in Chapter 3, the deficiency test, this means that your brain is either burning too much dopamine or not producing enough. Dopamine production determines your brain's power, which is measured as voltage. Voltage is the intensity with which the brain responds to a stimulus and the effectiveness of the brain's ability to process the information that monitors your physical and mental health. Without proper voltage you literally slow down and develop a dull edge.

As the power that drives your body's electrical output decreases, various symptoms and conditions can arise. The chart on the next page lists the various conditions that can occur as your body's electrical power—measured here in microvolts—begins to fail.

It is reasonable to assume that a dopamine deficiency will most likely occur in individuals who possess greater amounts of one of the other three biochemicals. By definition, any other nature has some relative dopamine lifestyle deficit. This does not mean that every dopamine deficiency must be corrected: each of us maintains our own healthy balance by the combination of all of the biochemicals. A minor deficiency may go unnoticed, or it can easily be addressed by following the lifestyle and diet suggestions in this chapter. A moderate or major deficiency requires immediate medical attention.

VOLTAGE	MEDICAL CONDITIONS
10–20	Normal to superior energy and concentration
9	Blues, mild hypertension, fatigue, mild memory loss or cognitive deficit
8	Insomnia, moderate hypertension, nicotine addiction, PMS, panic disorder, bipolar disorder
7	Obesity, moderate obsessive-compulsive disorder, mild depression, dysthymic disorder
6	Moderate addiction, major depression, various personality disorders, ischemia, severe vascular disorders
5	Toxic metal exposure, menopause, borderline personality disorder, chronic fatigue
4	Multiple sclerosis, problems related to dialysis, chronic depression, violence, tumors, diabetes, bypass surgery
3	Parkinson's disease, cirrhosis of the liver, multiple endocrine disorders
2	ADD, supranuclear palsy, Alzheimer's disease, disorders stemming from abnormal brain structure
1	Schizophrenia, cocaine abuse, HIV, hypoxia and other forms of oxygen deprivation, severe lead poisoning
0	Coma, severe metabolic encephalopathy, global brain disease

Dopamine natures can also develop a dopamine deficiency. These individuals are most likely to notice the smallest changes in their edge because they are most aware of how they feel when their dopamine is balanced. Dopamine natures will quickly notice when they feel less energetic and less powerful and when their thinking is not as sharp as they expect.

DOPAMINE-RELATED
SYMPTOMS AND CONDITIONS

With a dopamine deficiency, the early warning signs of deteriorating health are related to loss of energy: physically you experience fatigue, and mentally you're sluggish. These effects can show up in your body in a variety of ways and can affect any of the four major domains of brain function.

PHYSICAL ISSUES

Anemia

Balance problems

Blood sugar instability

Bone density loss

Carbohydrate binges

Constipation

Decreased desire for food

Decreased physical strength and activity

Diabetes

Diarrhea

Difficulty achieving orgasm

Digestion problems

Excessive sleep

Food cravings

Head and facial tremor

High blood pressure

Hyperglycemia

Inability to gain or lose weight

Joint pain

Kidney problems

Light-headedness

Low sex drive

Movement disorders

Narcolepsy

Nicotine cravings

Obesity

Parkinson's disease

Slow or poor metabolism

Slow or rigid movements

Substance abuse

Sugar or junk food cravings

Tension

Tremors

Thyroid disorders

Trouble swallowing

PERSONALITY ISSUES

Aggression

Anger

Carelessness

Depression

Fear of being observed

Guilt or feelings of worthlessness/ hopelessness

Hedonistic behavior

Inability to handle stress

Isolating oneself from others

Mood swings

Procrastination

Self-destructive thoughts

MEMORY ISSUES

Distractibility	Lack of working memory
Failure to listen and follow instructions	Poor abstract thinking
	Slow processing speed
Forgetfulness	

ATTENTION ISSUES

Attention deficit disorder	Hyperactivity
Decreased alertness	Impulsive behavior
Failure to finish tasks	Poor concentration

If you compare the above list with those that appear in the chapters on the other natures, you will find that some symptoms and conditions appear in more than one chapter. This repetition is caused by the binary nature of the neurotransmitters. While there are four primary neurotransmitters, they often work in similar ways. For example, both dopamine and acetylcholine act as the electrical on switch for the brain: they create energy the body uses for power and speed. On the other hand, GABA and serotonin are the electrical off switches: they create electricity necessary for calming the body and producing sleep. Because their functions are similar, similar symptoms may occur when either is deficient.

Also, the brain-mind-body connection has only a limited number of possible malfunctions. These malfunctions affect the rest of our system in similar ways. However, how a deficiency affects specific organs or systems varies by nature. For example, deficiencies in the dominant biochemical will produce issues concerning metabolism and food cravings in both dopamine and acetylcholine natures, yet a dopamine nature will crave carbohydrates and an acetylcholine nature will crave richer, fattier foods.

TYPICAL DOPAMINE DOMINOES

Obviously, no one person will have all of the listed symptoms of dopamine deficiency at once. Yet all of these symptoms are treated every day by thousands of doctors, most of whom overlook or may be unaware of the fact that they are caused by a dopamine deficiency. The value of the Edge Effect is in associating the earliest symptoms with a dopamine deficiency and showing you the easiest, least damaging, and most effective interventions.

Left unchecked, an unbalanced dopamine nature, or a dopamine deficiency for a different nature, can be the first sign of downward-spiraling health. Physical signs of dopamine deficiency might look like this: at first, your concentration may wander, your thinking and decision making may not be as quick as they once were, or your intensity at work might not be the same. You may find that it's taking more time and effort to get things done. You might sleep a little longer but still wake up tired. You grab coffee or caffeinated beverages more often than usual just to get you going. These supply the energy fix you need to feel like yourself, but the effect is temporary. So you reach for them continuously throughout the day, because otherwise you can't sustain your usual high level of performance.

You might be finding reasons to put off tasks instead of finishing them. You're distracted instead of focused, and you are not as tenacious or competitive as you used to be. You might gain weight or avoid social contact. You become more distant from significant others. In the evening, you may pour yourself a couple of drinks to settle down from the day's roller-coaster ride, not realizing that you are self-medicating to compensate for your dopamine deficiency, as well as the increased amount of coffee or other stimulants you might be taking. For the first time in your life, your sexual performance is compromised: you avoid sexual contact because you are just not interested. Every night you go to sleep thinking that by tomorrow you'll be back to normal. But tomorrow isn't any better. And neither is the next day. They bring more of the same: fatigue, loss of focus, agitation, diminished confidence concerning decisions and control of the future.

After a couple of years of struggling with these seemingly innocuous problems, you may be faced with symptoms and conditions that demand the attention of a medical professional. The weight gain was so gradual that you didn't realize how much you put on; now you're carrying around thirty extra pounds that you just can't seem to lose. Your blood pressure and cholesterol are elevated. The prescription drugs your doctor recommended, which at first you considered unnecessary, have become second nature to you. You no longer enjoy eating, thanks to irritable bowel syndrome or gastroesophageal reflux disorder. You deal with your health problems for a couple more years, until you come face-to-face with type II diabetes or kidney failure.

Although you might think this scenario is far-fetched, it represents what can happen when dopamine deficiency is left unchecked. If you can't recognize yourself in the above scenario, see if you can relate to the experiences of one of my patients, Joe.

When I first met Joe I wasn't sure he'd make it to a subsequent office visit: he was a prime candidate for a stroke. By the time this fifty-two-year-old came to see me, he was twenty-seven pounds overweight, and his blood pressure was slightly elevated even though he was on hypertension medication. He suffered from irritable and irregular bowels and gastro-esophageal reflux disorder, both of which frequently accompany hypertension. His cholesterol was 30 percent above normal. Joe was not sleeping well, and he felt tired all the time. His sex drive had decreased, which at least relieved his anxiety about his disappointing sexual performance.

Although Joe forced himself to work the same sixty-hour schedule he always did, he was not getting much done at the construction company he had started twenty years before. He wasn't able to stay focused at work and found himself just going through the motions. Joe was drinking numerous cups of coffee throughout the day simply to keep going. Normally cool under fire, Joe was losing his temper quite frequently, often for the most minor of reasons.

Joe no longer experienced satisfaction from anything. His meals were a chore because of an ongoing battle with his weight and digestive problems. And even though relationships had never been his strong suit, Joe's were becoming more strained every day. His second marriage was in trouble, and he found himself looking for reasons not to come home. When he found the time to see his two teenagers from his first marriage, their get-togethers always seemed to end in a screaming match.

Because Joe was a take-charge guy, he did try to relieve his symptoms. He had followed a number of diets and supplement programs to lose weight, but he was never able to keep the pounds from coming back. He took over-the-counter sleep aids but still woke up tired. Antacids were his constant companions. When his symptoms persisted beyond the help of these over-the-counter remedies, Joe visited his doctor.

The standard examination at the doctor's office revealed Joe's elevated blood pressure and cholesterol levels. A cardiac stress test came back normal—none of Joe's arteries were blocked. Prescriptions for hypertension, cholesterol, and gastroesophageal reflux disorder were written. Sleeping pills were also prescribed, to be taken as needed. Joe could use sildenafil (Viagra) whenever he wanted. He was put on a high-protein/low-carbohydrate diet and told to eat less.

After a month the gastroesophageal symptoms subsided, and Joe slept well on the nights he remembered to take his sleeping pill. But the fatigue persisted and may have actually worsened as a result of the blood pressure medications, which are known to slow down other internal systems. Joe tried to stick to the new diet, but it didn't appear that he'd lost any weight. He started to worry that he wasn't ever going to get better. When he called to voice his concerns, his doctor mentioned he might need an anti-anxiety medication. But adding yet another drug to his growing pharmacy just didn't seem right to Joe. That's when he visited me at one of my PATH Medical Centers.

THE STANDARD NONSTANDARD WORKUP

The PATH examination confirmed my first impression from our phone conference. After we identified Joe's dopamine-dominant nature, further examination revealed the underlying cause of Joe's complaints: his dopamine levels were dropping. His health restoration would have to start with balancing his nature.

Joe's patient history revealed a family background of hypertension, heart disease, and stroke, so genetic predisposition played a big part in Joe's health problems. But predisposition does not have to mean predetermination. Joe had always been attracted to the rush he'd experienced from using cocaine and Ecstasy when he was younger; unfortunately, these drugs had conditioned his brain to require other dopamine supplements, even years after he stopped using them. His ability to pay attention was inconsistent, his working memory score was low, and he could not quickly solve abstract problems. In short, his mind and his bodily functions were not sharp at all.

With conventional treatment approaches Joe's condition would have followed a predictable course: his blood pressure would push inexorably higher and become more difficult to manage, his cholesterol would continue to rise, his weight would slowly but surely increase. Sexual dysfunction would persist, even with pharmaceutical help: the frequency of his erections would decline from two or three per week to one every two or three weeks. All of these conditions would require higher doses of his current medications along with new medications, which would likely lead to complications, more symptoms, and more medications. With medications, caffeine, alcohol, and nicotine wreaking havoc with his internal chemistry, anxiety would become full-blown. Given Joe's weight gain, type II diabetes would be quite likely, with its attendant circulatory complications. Multiple coronary bypasses and/or angioplasties would only be a question of when—not if.

Fortunately for Joe, by learning about his nature and using all of the tools at his disposal to restore and maintain its balance, he turned his health around.

BALANCING YOUR DOPAMINE NATURE

Any dopamine deficiency can be corrected by using some combination of the seven treatment modalities: medications, hormones, supplements, diet, lifestyle, environment, and electrical treatments. The severity of your symptoms, however, will determine which type of treatment will work best for you. You can gauge the level of your deficiency by consulting the results of your deficiency test. A minor deficiency will range from 0 to 5; a moderate deficiency will range from 6 to 15; and a severe deficiency is considered anything over 15.

The following overview lists remedies for the most severe symptoms and conditions first, and progressively works down to treating minor deficiencies.

DOPAMINE-FRIENDLY MEDICATIONS

If you are experiencing severe dopamine-related symptoms, you can turn to certain pharmaceuticals that have been specifically designed to reverse a frontal lobe dopamine deficiency. These medications impact the body's adrenaline or energy system. Talk to your doctor regarding drug choices and specific doses that are right for you. Dosage will vary significantly based on your height, weight, and gender. Each of the following has properties that address a specific energy-deficient condition.

Allergies: pseudoephedrine (Sudafed), loratadine (Claritin)

Attention deficit disorder: methylphenidate (Ritalin), clonidine (Catapres), amphetamine (Adderall), atomoxetine (Strattera)

Cocaine abuse: bromocriptine (Parlodel), desipramine (Norpramin), clonidine (Catapres)

Depression: amphetamine (Adderall), venlafaxine (Effexor), bupropion (Wellbutrin), desipramine (Norpramin), nortriptyline (Pamelor), protriptyline (Vivactil), trimipramine (Surmontil)

Fatigue: venlafaxine (Effexor), desipramine (Norpramin), modafinil (Provigil)

Hypertension: guanfacine (Tenex), clonidine (Catapres)

Male sexual dysfunction: sildenafil (Viagra), vardenafil (Levitra), tadalafil (Cialis)

Narcolepsy: modafinil (Provigil), dextroamphetamine (Dexedrine)

Parkinson's disease: tolcapone (Tasmar), selegiline (Eldepryl), carbidopa-levodopa (Sinemet)

Tobacco abuse: bupropion (Wellbutrin), venlafaxine (Effexor)

Treatment-resistant depression: amphetamine (Adderall), dextro-amphetamine (Dexedrine), methylphenidate (Ritalin, Concerta)

Weight loss: phentermine (Ionamin), diethylpropion (Tenuate), phendimetrazine (Prelu), sibutramine (Meridia)

Once you have balanced your dopamine by following the suggestions in the rest of this chapter, you should not need these serious medications. But until your dopamine is balanced, you may require some combination of these prescription drugs. Some of these drugs directly affect dopamine production, while others merely treat symptoms so that you can get a jump start toward better health.

The art of medicine is in correctly diagnosing a condition and prescribing the pharmaceutical that is most appropriate for it. As your condition improves, you can slowly discontinue these medications, and possibly replace them with natural supplements. However, all issues related to prescription medications must be resolved in consultation with a medical doctor.

HORMONES

Each of the four primary neurotransmitters has a characteristic hormone associated with it. When a particular biochemical becomes deficient, this hormone comes in to take its place. For example, the body naturally increases production of cortisol when there is a dopamine imbalance. Made in the adrenal glands, cortisol regulates blood pressure and cardiovascular function as well as the body's use of proteins, carbohydrates, and fats. Cortisol is the backup adrenaline hormone, so that when you are under stress, your cortisol levels increase. Your pulse quickens, you become red-faced, and your blood pressure goes up.

It is also true that as we age, we lose the ability to produce hormones in the amounts and rates required for optimal health. When these drop-offs occur we must supplement our own hormone levels. While the hormones listed below are necessary to enhance any nature, a dopamine nature will notice more readily when they require supplementation. Human growth hormone (HGH) is available in injectable form and is very expensive. A less expensive alternative is to augment existing HGH with amino acid products such as creatine and arginine. All of the following natural hormones help increase voltage and provide energy to the brain. They also have other specific functions. As with prescription medications, all issues related to hormone replacement must be addressed in conjunction with a medical doctor.

Bone building: calcitonin (Miacalcin)

Increases sex drive: testosterone

Fights fatigue: DHEA (dehydroepiandrosterone)

Builds heart blood vessels, and memory: vasopressin

Prevents loss of bone mass: human growth hormone (HGH), testosterone

Increases concentration: thyroid combination treatment, which includes thyroxine (T4) and triiodothyronine (T3), also known as pathroid

Increases muscle tone: human growth hormone (HGH), somatostatin

Elevates mood: thyroxine

Treats sugar deficiencies: insulin, growth hormone (insulin growth factors)

Treats sugar deficiencies under stress: glucagon, cortisol

Maintains skin, hair, teeth, circulation: estrogen

Restores kidney function: erythropoietin

Addresses gastrointestinal absorption issues: cholecystokinin

Replenishes hormones when under stress: cortisol

Blood vessel and inflammatory disorders: prostaglandin

DIET

For many conditions—especially those present in the early stages of deficiency—you may not need a doctor's help to restore your dopamine imbalance. You can take matters into your own hands by following the nature-balancing suggestions for your diet and supplement regimen.

Making healthy dietary choices is the foundation for a stable nature—one that will support you for your entire lifetime. The easiest and most natural way for you to keep your dopamine nature balanced involves the choices you make when you eat.

SOLVING CHRONIC OBESITY

Rapid and significant weight gain is one of the hallmarks of a dopamine deficiency. Obesity, a burgeoning condition that is defined as 20 percent above ideal body weight, is one of the great health problems Americans are facing today. Ideal weight is determined as 5 pounds for every inch over five feet for women, and 6 pounds for every inch over five feet for men, starting at 106 pounds. While most doctors recognize that obesity is a metabolic disorder, they might miss the point that metabolism is governed by dopamine. Under the right program, dopamine-deficient patients can lose their excess weight and keep it off for good.

I have seen hundreds of patients for issues of significant weight gain. I'm happy to say that many of my patients have been successful in their battle. Most have followed a dopamine-balancing regimen, which includes a program that combines supplements, natural hormones, and conventional medicine. Many have lost more than 150 pounds.

Using the Edge Effect to increase your dopamine is a good strategy when you are trying to lose weight. You might notice that highly stimulated people are usually thin or have the ability to lose weight quickly. This is because they have high-dopamine natures. The more dopamine you produce, the faster your metabolism works, which makes it possible for you to burn calories more efficiently.

If you have a dopamine deficiency and follow the suggestions below, you might experience weight loss as you learn to eat healthier foods. You can select dopamine-producing foods that will increase your metabolism and boost your dopamine Edge Effect. When you do so, the occasional pizza, pasta, or other treats with which you sometimes indulge yourself will have no harmful effect at all. When your dopamine is balanced, you will not crave sugars and carbohydrates. Your increased energy will also make you want to get out and exercise more, which will help you lose weight faster.

NUTRIENTS THAT RAISE YOUR DOPAMINE LEVELS

Nature-specific diets are not weight loss diets. They are not about portion control, counting calories, or focusing on a particular nutrient group such as proteins, fats, or carbohydrates. Instead, the following are lists of dietary choices you can make to boost your levels of dopamine and eventually help your brain create more dopamine on its own.

The goal of a dopamine diet is to ensure that the body has enough raw materials for a steady supply of tyrosine and phenylalanine, two amino acids that are precursors to dopamine. These amino acids are found in many protein-rich foods.

Be sure to round out a high-protein meal with lots of additional fruits and vegetables, even if they don't appear on the lists in this chapter. You may also drink any nonalcoholic, sugar-free beverage you prefer, ideally noncarbonated so it won't produce gas. Caffeinated beverages happen to be good for dopamine-deficient people. If, however, you are serotonin deficient, caffeine could give you insomnia. GABA-deficient types might react with nervousness and palpitations; for the acetylcholine deficient, caffeine can contribute to jumpiness and the inability to think clearly.

Phenylalanine: Fatigue and Pain Reliever

Phenylalanine is an essential amino acid found in the brain and blood plasma that can convert in the body to tyrosine, which in turn is used to synthesize dopamine. Sources of phenylalanine are high-protein foods such as meat, cottage cheese, and wheat germ. Phenylalanine can also be found in the sugar substitute aspartame, which is sold under the brand names NutraSweet and Equal. These artificial sweeteners have no calories, do not affect blood sugar, and are generally safe. However, they should be avoided entirely by those who have phenylketonuria. Pregnant or lactating women should always seek the advice of their doctor regarding the use of artificial sweeteners.

Increasing your phenylalanine levels can be effective for treating mild depression, and particularly in countering fatigue. In my office, I have found that about 10 to 50 percent of depressed patients have low plasma phenylalanine, and eating phenylalanine-rich foods is an effective treatment. Your body can elevate levels of phenylalanine in times of infection or fatigue. Phenylalanine levels are lowered by increased caffeine ingestion.

An average adult ingests 4 grams of phenylalanine per day, and may optimally need up to 6 grams daily through supplementation. Use the food list on the following page as needed.

Tyrosine: Dopamine Builder

When phenylalanine is converted to tyrosine, this amino acid increases resistance to stress and acts as one of the body's natural pain relievers. As mentioned above, tyrosine is used to synthesize dopamine. It also builds norepinephrine, which is chemically related to adrenaline; tyrosine can give dopamine-deficient people the increased energy they are lacking. Foods that contain high amounts of tyrosine include chicken, duck, cottage cheese, and wheat germ.

THE DOPAMINE DIET: PHENYLALANINE IN FOODS

FOOD	AMOUNT	CONTENT (G)
Chicken	6–8 oz	1.60
Chocolate (dark)	2–4 oz.	0.40
Cottage cheese	1 cup	1.70
Duck	6–8 oz.	1.60
Egg	1	0.35
Granola	1 cup	0.65
Low-fat, low-salt cheeses	1 oz.	0.35
Luncheon meat	6–8 oz	1.10
Oat flakes or rolled oats	1 cup	0.50
Pork	6–8 oz.	1.30
Ricotta	1 cup	1.35
Sausage meat	6–8 oz.	0.50
Soybeans	6–8 oz.	1.20
Turkey	6–8 oz.	1.60
Walnuts	6–8 oz.	1.40
Wheat germ	1 cup	1.35
Whole milk	1 cup	0.40
Wild game	6–8 oz	2.60
Yogurt (plain, nonfat)	1 cup	0.40

Physicians at Harvard Medical School have pioneered the use of a daily dose of up to 6 grams of tyrosine to decrease symptoms of medication-resistant depression with good results. Tyrosine creates so much raw energy that in extremely large doses (i.e., greater than 20 grams daily), it can reduce your appetite. However, low doses have a less consistent effect. The minimum daily tyrosine requirement is about 1,000 mg. for an average adult. Use the food list at right to increase your total tyrosine consumption in order to balance your dopamine deficiency.

DOPAMINE-BOOSTING DIET

If your dopamine nature has been diminishing, or if you are trying to enhance this biochemical to complement another nature, try the diet on page 86. These menus span three days and can give you an idea of foods you can eat that will increase your dopamine. How often you

THE DOPAMINE DIET: TYROSINE IN FOODS

FOOD	AMOUNT	CONTENT (G)
Chicken	6–8 oz.	0.40
Chocolate	1 cup	0.40
Cottage cheese	1 cup	1.70
Duck	6–8 oz.	0.60
Egg	1	0.25
Granola	1 cup	0.40
Oat flakes or rolled oats	1 cup	0.35
Pork	6–8 oz.	1.20
Ricotta	1 cup	1.50
Turkey	6–8 oz.	0.70
Wheat germ	1 cup	1.00
Whole milk	1 cup	0.40
Wild game	6–8 oz.	1.50
Yogurt	1 cup	0.40

repeat this diet depends on your deficiency level. If you have a minor deficiency, then you should follow a three-day course once a month. If you have a moderate deficiency, you should follow this three-day course once a week. An extreme deficiency requires at least six days a week of this specific diet.

The main component of this high-protein, low-fat regimen is foods that are rich in phenylalanine and tyrosine.

DEFICIENCY CRAVINGS

If you are experiencing a dopamine deficiency, you might find yourself bingeing on sweets or caffeine. Both provide the energy boost that you might feel you are lacking. While these foods will certainly work in the short term, the long-range consequences can be devastating. Too much coffee can make you jittery and irritable, as well as produce irregular heartbeat. Too much sugar can lead to rapid weight gain, as well as type 2 diabetes, where your body can no longer balance the ratio between insulin and sugar.

If you want to offset your dopamine deficiency, you must eliminate processed sugars and baked goods made with refined white flour from

---

DAY 1

BREAKFAST   2 soft-boiled or poached eggs with 4 oz. spinach and 1 clove of raw garlic; add some seasonings for flavor (no seasoning is off-limits). Finish with a cup of iced green tea with lemon and Equal.

LUNCH   4–6 oz. sardines with 6 oz. soybeans, almonds, and cranberries. Add 1–2 tablespoons olive oil–balsamic vinegar dressing and some seasonings. Finish with iced tea with lemon and Equal.

DINNER   6–8 oz. lamb (seasoned with herbs) with 6 oz. brown rice and 6 oz. (total) of mixed grilled asparagus, carrots, and onions. For dessert, 2 oz. berries mixed in ½ cup plain yogurt. Finish with cranberry tea.

DAY 2

BREAKFAST   2-egg omelet with 2 oz. roasted turkey and fresh radishes. Finish with coffee with cinnamon.

LUNCH   6 oz. light tuna mixed with olive oil to taste on 1 slice whole-wheat bread with lettuce, tomatoes, and onions. Finish with 6 oz. freshly squeezed grapefruit juice.

DINNER   6 oz. salad of beets and apples with 2 oz. goat cheese and balsamic vinegar (no olive oil). One grilled Cajun-spiced chicken breast and 4 oz. (total) of mixed steamed snow peas, red beans, and corn. Finish with ginger tea.

---

your diet as much as possible, and reduce caffeinated beverages to no more than two cups per day. For some dopamine-related physical illnesses, you might want to eliminate foods high in saturated fat if you need to reduce your cholesterol, and carbohydrate restriction can help you lose weight and reduce fatigue.

DAY 3

BREAKFAST	2 oz. sardines with dark green lettuce and 1 cup plain yogurt with 2 oz. mixed berries, almonds, and walnuts. Finish with Earl Grey tea.
LUNCH	6 oz. baked salmon on a 6 oz. garden salad with olive oil and vinegar with a few whole-wheat or rice crackers. Finish with green tea.
DINNER	4–6 oz. lean steak or veal with 4 oz. steamed green beans, toasted almonds, and cranberries. Finish with a cup of oolong tea.
HEALTHY SNACKS	2 oz. cottage cheese with grapes ½ cup plain yogurt with blueberries 1 soft-boiled egg with some baby carrots 1 green apple with 2 tablespoons of almonds

---

By increasing your consumption of phenylalanine and tyrosine, you can restore your dopamine to optimal levels. Your body will be getting the energy it needs from these amino acids—not from sugar and caffeine. You will find that you are no longer craving foods that will give you energy, because your body will be producing enough on its own. Changing your dietary habits is not easy, but the benefits of your dopamine diet will be evident after a few weeks. Your energy level will rise, your concentration and thinking will sharpen, and your sleep will be more restful. Over time, you will likely be able to eliminate medications for digestion and sleep.

VITAMINS AND SUPPLEMENTS

Taking readily available vitamins and supplements is an excellent way to ensure a steady supply of dopamine-friendly nutrients. Because they are energy-related, they are best taken on a full stomach after you've eaten breakfast or lunch—you wouldn't want an extra charge in the evening when it's time to relax.

DOPAMINE BOOSTERS FOR BRAIN ENERGY
(SUGGESTED DAILY SUPPLEMENTAL DOSES)

	Minor Deficit (0–5)	Moderate Deficit (6–15)	Severe Deficit (15+)
Phenylalanine	500 mg.	1,000 mg.	1,000–2,000 mg.
Tyrosine	500 mg.	1,000 mg.	1,000–2,000 mg.
Methionine	250 mg.	500 mg.	1,000 mg.
Rhodiola	50 mg.	100 mg.	200 mg.
Pyridoxine	5 mg.	10 mg.	50 mg.
B complex	25 mg.	50 mg.	100 mg.
Phosphatidylserine	50 mg.	100 mg.	200 mg.
Ginkgo biloba	50 mg.	75 mg.	100 mg.

Each of the primary neurotransmitters has a nutrient precursor, and dopamine is derived from the amino acids phenylalanine and tyrosine. Phenylalanine is made first, and then gets converted into tyrosine. When we are healthy, our diet usually provides adequate quantities of these natural substances. However, when the first symptoms of illness occur, these nutrients can be supplemented to avoid more serious conditions. Therefore, augmenting these amino acids becomes your first line of defense to regain wellness and increase your Edge Effect.

For example, the supplement D, L-phenylalanine can be an effective pain reliever and antidepressant with many potential therapeutic benefits. D, L-phenylalanine inhibits enkephalinase enzyme, which breaks down the body's endogenous opioids. It can be used to lessen the symptoms of PMS and Parkinson's disease. Phenylalanine is better absorbed than tyrosine and may cause fewer headaches. However, in order for phenylalanine to be properly metabolized, you will need sufficient quantities of biopterin, a form of folic acid; iron, niacin, vitamin B_6, copper, and vitamin C must also be ingested.

L-dopa, which is used in the treatment for Parkinson's disease, is made from tyrosine. It can be also be used as a safe and lasting therapy for hypotension, ventricular fibrillation, and appetite suppression. Drugs that prolong the effects of tyrosine have been used as aphrodisiacs, including sildenafil (Viagra). Large doses of tyrosine supplements such as yohimbine may stimulate sex drive (and may raise blood pressure). Tyrosine supplement therapy may also be useful in treating drug addiction, temporarily replacing cocaine and amphetamines much the way methadone replaces heroin for addicts. Folic acid, copper, and vitamin C are nutrients necessary for these reactions to occur.

I have developed a unique dopamine supplement formula (see table on opposite page), which I call Brain Energy. It contains thiamine, tyrosine, phenylalanine, low-dose caffeine, folic acid, and chromium. Taken on a daily basis, this supplement can help to build your metabolism. This specific formula helps keep your edge sharp and decreases symptoms of fatigue, light-headedness, weight gain, and diminished libido. Taking the supplements listed at left, in the amounts indicated, will increase your energy and return your attention to its former levels of excellence.

Dopaminergic symptoms and conditions are best treated with specific supplements. The recommended daily allowance, or RDA, for each is in parentheses:

Diminished sex drive: yohimbine (15–20 mg.)

Fatigue: chromium (men 35 mcg., women 25 mcg.), guarana (200–2,000 mg.)

Impotence: arginine (has an effect similar to Viagra) (1,000–10,000 mg.)

Inflammation: fish oil (1,000–3,000 mg.), aspirin (1,200–1,500 mg. for a short period of time), and willow bark (200–1,000 mg.)

Narcolepsy: guarana (1,000–2,000 mg.)

Substance abuse: thiamine (men 1.5 mg., women 1.1 mg.)

Treatment-resistant depression: Rhodiola rosea (50–750 mg.)

Weight loss: hydroxycitric acid (500–1,500 mg.), conjugated linoleic acid (2,000–3,000 mg.)

LIFESTYLE

The risk for dopamine natures of leading a high-energy lifestyle is burning out the brain's power supply of dopamine faster than it can be replenished. Rather than using quick fixes such as sugar and caffeine, it is far healthier to balance high energy output with regular periods of relaxation and restoration. Dopamine natures are used to handling stress, but everyone needs to take a break now and then, especially if you are experiencing a dopamine deficiency. Here are some examples of stress-busting activities that need to be incorporated into your day so that the brain can resynchronize and rebalance to produce more dopamine.

EXERCISE: ALTERNATE DEEP BREATHING

Deep breathing exercises are ideal for the person with a primary dopamine nature. These can slow your body down and provide a feeling of peace, which rests the brain while it's awake. They will help you create more energy and at the same time embrace a feeling of complete relaxation and peace of mind.

Sit quietly in a comfortable position and take five slow, deep breaths.

Exhale all your air completely, and then seal off your right nostril with your thumb, completely filling your lungs through your left nostril.

Use your ring finger or pinkie to seal off the other nostril, so that both are closed. Hold your breath for fifteen seconds. Release your right nostril and exhale.

Inhale again through your right nostril, seal off both nostrils, and hold your breath for another fifteen seconds. Release your left nostril and exhale.

Complete this exercise three times, then relax, sit quietly, and take five complete breaths through both nostrils.

OTHER LIFESTYLE STRATEGIES

For half an hour each day, try to set aside the time for quiet relaxation, which can include non-work-related reading, watching nonviolent television programs, or even playing a competitive game such as chess.

Anaerobic exercise, such as weight lifting, should be done three times per week. Use weights that involve an exertion of effort to do ten to fifteen repetitions for each exercise, then increase the weights when the repetitions become easy. You might want to work with a personal trainer who can develop a personal weight-training program for you.

ENVIRONMENT

Exposure to lead from old paint, leaking batteries, or solder (molten lead used to fasten metal) has been proven to reduce the brain's dopamine supply. Read warning labels carefully and wear a protective mask in order to protect your dopamine balance if you absolutely must be around lead-based products.

Cadmium from cigarette smoke also decreases dopamine. If you smoke, now is the time to quit: there are really no more excuses for continuing this extremely unhealthy habit. Thousands of smokers have broken this addiction with our dopamine nutrient supplements. If you don't smoke and find yourself near smokers, move as far away as possible.

GETTING INTO BALANCE

Nature-based treatment is not miraculous, it's just good medicine. Getting to the source of an illness by discovering your nature is the path to health. With my patient Joe, the key wasn't his weight, his digestive system, his hypertension, or his cholesterol. Continued treatment of these isolated symptoms would have just resulted in new ones. The real solution to Joe's myriad health problems was balancing his dopamine and bringing back his edge.

Obviously, Joe couldn't lose his extra weight overnight. Nor could he lower his blood pressure and cholesterol levels rapidly. But we could do something right away about his gastroesophageal reflux disorder and his energy level. When we replaced his gastroesophageal reflux disorder medication with licorice root and had him sleep with his head elevated, Joe's symptoms disappeared within a week. That immediately improved his sleeping pattern, which is critical to having the brain restore itself. You know what you can accomplish in an eight-hour day; the brain actually does far more with an eight-hour night.

After ten days of restful sleep and taking DHEA, HGH, and the

Brain Energy formula, Joe started to feel his old energy returning. His anxiety symptoms disappeared after two weeks. Taking care of Joe's digestion and improving his sleep and sex drive did wonders for improving his whole attitude. When his energy returned to normal after the first month, he started to feel competent again at work. Joe's recovery was really picking up steam. Then other parts of his treatment program began to do their part as well.

The HGH, which reduced Joe's carbohydrate cravings, and his dopamine diet began to show results after the first month: Joe lost nine pounds in four weeks and was able to keep them off since he no longer craved sweets and simple carbohydrates. Because he was totally committed to restoring his health, he took a hard look at how he lived every day, and made some changes he felt he could sustain. Probably the most important thing he did was assess his priorities so that his overall stress level could be ratcheted down a couple of notches. Work would always be important, but not everything had to be done yesterday. He established new routines in other parts of his life, and he made sure to include a routine of gym visits, breaks in the park, and deep breathing exercises.

After three months, Joe was off all prescription medications. He had lost twenty-seven pounds and was able to maintain this loss. His blood pressure was back to normal, he had no signs of gastroesophageal reflux disorder, his energy was restored, his sex drive was good, and he was no longer considering a second divorce. That was two years ago. Today Joe is maintaining normal weight, is physically fit, and is retaining his strategic thinking and concentration abilities. He's calm and stable, and his relationships are on an even keel.

5

THE CREATIVE
ACETYLCHOLINE NATURE

IF YOU SCORED HIGH on the Braverman Nature Assessment for acetylcholine, your brain chemistry is dominated by this neurotransmitter, which is produced in the brain's parietal lobes. The parietal lobes are responsible for thinking functions, such as comprehension of language, intelligence, and attention.

In this chapter you will learn about your acetylcholine nature and see how it affects all areas of your physical and mental health. More important, you will be able to point to some of the specific ailments you might be experiencing and learn how to correct them by addressing an acetylcholine deficiency. By doing so you will be taking the first step to better health.

THE ACETYLCHOLINE NATURE
PERSONALITY PROFILE

People with an acetylcholine nature are adept at working with their senses and view the world in sensory terms. They are highly creative and open to new ideas. If you have an acetylcholine nature, you represent 17 percent of the world's population. You are a quick thinker who is constantly taking others into consideration. This nature is devoted to making something the best it can be, no matter how much effort it requires. Your flexibility, creativity, and impulsivity open you up to try anything as long as it offers the promise of excitement and introduces you to something new.

A balanced acetylcholine nature is intuitive and innovative. You take pleasure in anything involving words, ideas, and communication, and are able to share your enthusiasm with others. This nature makes for ideal counselors, mediators, think tank members, yoga and meditation instructors, religious leaders, and members of public-service organizations. Brain speed impacts the creative function, so artists, writers, advertising professionals, and actors are all likely to be acetylcholine dominant. An educator with an acetylcholine nature would gravitate toward teaching art or literature; an accountant would gravitate toward specializing in forecasting and projections; a plumber might find himself teaching in a trade school.

If you're acetylcholine dominant, you're extremely sociable, even charismatic. You love meeting and greeting, and making new friends. You come across to others as being authentic and grounded. Relationships come easily to you, and others find you charming. You invest a great deal of energy in all of your relationships—at work, in the community, and at home—and feel that you are personally reaping the rewards. An eternal optimist, you envision the possibilities in everyone. You are attentive to the needs of your children and romantic with your significant other. You possess a unique ability to remember other people's feelings and reactions, which enables you to avoid hurting them. Thanks to your altruism and benevolence, you are quite popular with a broad range of people.

Adventure is your hallmark. You are always open to trying new things and are not afraid of failure. Travel is exciting, yet you can also thrive by staying home and reading about the lives and experiences of others. Your quest for learning makes you interested in a variety of topics and adept at sharing your knowledge with others.

The Edge Effect occurs when you've maximized your acetylcholine nature. These are the times when your thinking is crystal clear and you are formulating new ideas about the world around you. You might be creating something artistic, or you might be deeply involved in your spiritual practice. Or perhaps you're motivating others to become the best they can be.

TOO MUCH ACETYLCHOLINE

It is possible, however, to have too much of a good thing. People with acetylcholine natures who produce excessive amounts of this biochemical are at risk when they give too much of themselves to others, to the point of becoming masochistic. Individuals who produce an overabundance of acetylcholine might feel the world is taking advantage of them, or they may become paranoid. Too much acetylcholine can drive an individual into isolation.

OUT OF BALANCE:
ACETYLCHOLINE DEFICIENCY

If you scored high for acetylcholine in the second test in Chapter 3, then you are acetylcholine deficient. An acetylcholine deficiency occurs when your brain is either burning too much acetylcholine or not producing enough. Acetylcholine regulates your ability to process sensory input and access stored information. First, input comes to the brain as a global response to sensory stimuli, including touch, taste, smell, vision, and sound. This information is processed into memories and thoughts, which are then stored in your brain and used as the basis of your knowledge.

Your response to sensory stimuli is measured by your brain's speed. Acetylcholine, displayed as alpha waves, controls your brain speed by determining the rate at which electrical signals are processed throughout your body, literally connecting your body's physical experiences to memories and thoughts. This electrical rate is one of the factors that determine your brain's real, or functional, age which may be very different from your chronological age, depending on your brain's health. When your brain speed slows, the brain doesn't have time to connect all the new stimuli to previously stored information before the next batch of stimuli rolls in; some information winds up getting discarded before it's processed, so recall starts to become spotty. You cannot react to sensory stimuli as fast as you used to. This causes forgetfulness, because your brain can't connect new stimuli to previously stored memories or thoughts. Also, slowed impulses to the body result in organs functioning less well. When this occurs, you might feel like you are losing your edge.

The chart on the following page shows how physical and mental changes relate to changes in electrical brain speed, measured in milliseconds. At the beginning of the chart please note that too much of a good thing—in this case brain speed—can cause its own special problems. As brain speed dips below normal, a different set of issues comes into play. When you lose just seven milliseconds of brain speed, you can recognize that your thinking is slowing down, even if your baseline is much faster than average.

SPEED (MILLISECONDS)	MEDICAL CONDITIONS
275 High Acetylcholine	Speeds this high typically indicate overstimulation due to cocaine or amphetamines
280	Panic disorder, manic episodes of bipolar disorder, anxiety
290	Anxiety or normal, depending on age
300	Normal
310	Normal
320	Normal
330	hyperthyroidism, post-traumatic stress disorder, mild hypertension, learning difficulties
340	Fatigue, hyperlipidemia, mild anemia, hypothyroidism, obesity
350	Attention deficit disorder, narcolepsy, menopause, diabetes, coronary artery disease, chronic obstructive pulmonary disease, cancer, uncontrolled or poorly controlled hypertension
360	Congestive heart failure, moderate anemia, learning disorders
370	Multiple sclerosis, HIV, encephalopathy, dementia associated with medical disease, seizure disorder, epilepsy, severe anemia
380	Parkinson's disease, schizophrenia, kidney failure, head injury

SPEED (MILLISECONDS)	MEDICAL CONDITIONS
390	Multiple system atrophy, stroke, supranuclear palsy
400	Early-stage Alzheimer's disease and other dementias
420 Low acetylcholine	Severe Alzheimer's and other dementias

It is reasonable to assume that an acetylcholine deficiency will most likely occur in individuals who possess greater amounts of one of the other three biochemicals. By definition, most other natures are somewhat acetylcholine-deficient. This does not mean that any acetylcholine deficiency must be corrected: each of us maintains our own healthy balance through the combination of all of the biochemicals. A minor deficiency may go unnoticed or can easily be corrected by following the lifestyle and diet suggestions in this chapter. A moderate or major deficiency, however, requires immediate medical attention.

Acetylcholine natures can also develop an acetylcholine deficiency, which is usually experienced as a keen awareness that they are not quite themselves. These individuals are most likely to notice the smallest changes in their edge because they are most aware of how they feel when their acetylcholine is balanced. Acetylcholine natures will quickly notice when they can't remember things as easily as they used to.

ACETYLCHOLINE-RELATED SYMPTOMS AND CONDITIONS

For those with an acetylcholine nature, or others who are experiencing an acetylcholine deficiency, the early warning signs of deteriorating health are related to loss of thought: physically you experience sensory loss, and mentally you've lost your enthusiasm for life and may become forgetful. The brain is the generator of half of the body's energy signals. When the brain slows down, so does the entire body. This can show up in your body in a variety of ways and can affect any of the four major domains of brain function.

PHYSICAL ISSUES

Agitation
Alzheimer's disease
Anxiety
Arthritis
Autism
Cholesterol elevation
Decline in sexual ability
Diabetes
Difficulty urinating
Dry cough
Dry mouth
Dyslexia
Excessive or frequent urination
Eye disorders
Fat cravings

Frequent bowel movements
Glaucoma
Hypoarousal
Inability to carry out motor
  commands
Inability to recognize objects
Inflammatory disorders
Involuntary movements
Multiple sclerosis
Osteoporosis
Reading/writing disorders
Rigidity or flaccidity
Slowness of movement
Speech problems

PERSONALITY ISSUES

Bipolar disorder
Calculation errors
Changes in personality and
  language

Hysterical behavior
Mood swings
Rule breaking

MEMORY ISSUES

Learning disorders
Loss of immediate visual and
  verbal memory

Memory disturbance
Memory lapses

ATTENTION ISSUES

Attention problems
Difficulty concentrating
Diminished comprehension

Impaired abstract thinking and
  judgment
Impaired creativity

Of all the natures, brain functional impairment due to deficiency is most apparent in acetylcholine natures. Yet diagnoses are often made and treatments recommended without an adequate assessment of the neurotransmitter responsible for these symptoms. The value of *The Edge*

Effect is in properly associating these symptoms with an acetylcholine deficiency and providing you with information about the easiest, least damaging, and most effective interventions.

If you compare the lists at left with those that appear in the text on other natures, you will find that some symptoms and conditions appear more than once. This repetition is caused by the binary nature of the four major neurotransmitters, with both dopamine and acetylcholine acting as the electrical on switch for the brain, and GABA and serotonin as the electrical off switches. Because their functions are similar, similar symptoms may occur when either is deficient.

Also, the brain-mind-body connection has only a limited number of possible malfunctions, so these malfunctions affect the rest of our system in similar ways. However, how a deficiency affects specific organs or systems varies by nature. For example, while acetylcholine and dopamine deficiencies both lead to attention issues, dopamine-related deficiencies cause a loss of the energy to learn, while acetylcholine deficiencies actually lead to forgetfulness.

ACETYLCHOLINE DOMINOES

Left unchecked, an unbalanced acetylcholine nature, or an acetylcholine deficiency in a different nature, can lead to a slide in your health. Instead of constantly seeking out human interaction, you find yourself avoiding contact with others. There is a noticeable tension in your relationships that wasn't there before. Order, schedules, and routines—never strong suits for you—become totally out of hand, and you can't manage your daily schedule. Where you used to move rapidly from one idea to another, from one activity to another, from one person to another, now you start to obsess about what should come next.

Physically, muscles and bones ache, but not the same ones all the time—and you can't seem to pinpoint one particular area. For the first time in your life, you're not enjoying sex, because of vaginal dryness or an inability to sustain an erection. While you don't have trouble falling asleep, you find yourself waking up an hour before your alarm clock goes off. You find solace in comfort foods such as heavy home-style meals, fried foods, and ice cream.

Months later, physical changes are harder to ignore. You're several pounds overweight. Those elusive muscle and joint aches are still with you, and other, more disconcerting symptoms appear: your visual perception is off, and your reflexes are slower. You can't remember the names of people you just met. You can't seem to formulate a plan of action. Drawing conclusions and making decisions require new effort.

Because you are open-minded, you might visit a number of alternative healers. A chiropractor adjusts your back, and an acupuncturist short-circuits your various aches and pains. A massage therapist relaxes you, at least temporarily. While you do feel better, the results never last. The physical symptoms don't disappear; they just hibernate for a while. Your mood swings are more pronounced, and you seem to be staying in the low periods longer than ever.

Your medical doctor gives you a physical exam and is nonplussed by the results. Other than your being a little overweight—which was obvious—the doctor doesn't uncover anything to explain your condition. She tells you to watch what you eat and to exercise, and that you might be experiencing anxiety. She writes a prescription for Prozac, which you take, but your symptoms never go away.

After months of effort, your diet has not worked. Your cravings for fried food and ice cream are still with you. You can't remember much of anything anymore—you can't even remember to make notes. You don't want to go to work, and you don't want to run into anyone you know. You may experience a series of accidents, such as falling off a ladder, tripping on a sidewalk crack, and wrecking your car. You no longer care about people or want to be with them. And physical deterioration can occur in tandem with cognitive failures—muscle and bone aches are constant, and simply walking becomes difficult. You are finally diagnosed with osteoporosis combined with arthritic inflammation. A deficit of acetylcholine slows bone preservation as calcium leaks out of the bones, which can be a contributing factor in arthritis, hardening of the arteries, loss of attention functions, Alzheimer's disease, and other dementias.

Although you might think this scenario is far-fetched, it is exactly what can happen when an acetylcholine deficiency is left unchecked. If you can't recognize yourself in the above scenario, see if you can relate to the experiences of my patient Nancy. At fifty-five, she had spent the past twenty years building a successful psychology practice by connecting well with her patients. She was highly skilled at pointing out different ways of seeing things and at making alternative solutions available so that patients could help themselves. But she was clueless about helping herself.

For more than a year, Nancy ignored or put up with her symptoms. She thought that her weight gain and her conflicts with her husband and children were due to mood swings caused by menopause. What most annoyed her were the memory lapses that had progressed from an occasional inconvenience to a daily occurrence. She couldn't remember a patient's history without reviewing the chart, which previously she had rarely needed to do. She wasn't thinking clearly, and she was no longer confident in her professional expertise. Plagued with the thought that someone would discover her lapses, she considered closing her practice.

Physically, Nancy was experiencing odd and varied symptoms. Her muscles ached; at first it was just a sporadic annoyance, but soon it progressed to a daily problem. She knew older people often have trouble getting around, but to have pain merely when she walked seemed a bit premature. Worse, sexual relations were also becoming painful because of vaginal dryness. Combined with her weight gain and her thinning hair, she felt that she was not attractive to her husband, and she began to withdraw from him physically and emotionally.

Nancy was mired in a low mood most of the time. She was bored by her patients during sessions and was terrified that they would find out. She was barely involved with her three children—a high school senior, a college sophomore, and a newlywed. She just didn't seem to have the energy or desire to be engaged in their lives, even though each was on the cusp of something new and exciting. The thought of being a grandmother, which she had constantly talked about with eager anticipation, was now a source of dread for her. Uninterested in her patients, uninvolved with her children, and distant from her husband, Nancy found herself alone most of the time.

As a health care professional, Nancy was aware of the efficacy of alternative treatments for many conditions. But when six months of visits to an acupuncturist, a massage therapist, and a nutritionist made no impact on her conditions, Nancy visited her primary care physician. From the doctor's point of view, complications associated with menopause explained quite a lot. Nancy's hormones were certainly in a state of flux, and this was a contributing factor to her depression, which in turn played a role in her weight gain, fatigue, and low mood. She was given a prescription for Premarin—a natural, but not bioidentical estrogen. (Premarin is derived from female horses.) Her doctor assured her this would address her vaginal dryness, her hair loss, and her low mood. Paxil, an antidepressant, would also help her out of her doldrums. Tenuate—a prescription stimulant—would give her an energy boost to counteract her recent lethargy. When all of these kicked in, her doctor explained, her memory would recover. But Nancy was also informed that her cholesterol was 50 percent higher than normal—she would need a prescription for Lipitor to get this under control. And the extra weight? Her doctor put her on a strict diet—1,500 calories per day— and warned her to stay away from fats.

Nancy's doctor was confident she would be fine. Yet four months later Nancy was still waiting to get better despite her best efforts. She followed her diet religiously and dropped fifteen pounds, but she felt hungry all the time and resented not being able to eat what she wanted. Nancy was able to engage with her children, but she still wasn't motivated to be closer to her husband, though her ability to have intercourse improved. Perhaps worst of all, there was no sign of improvement in her memory, and her practice continued to suffer. When, on top of everything else, she started to have difficulties sleeping, she showed up in my office.

Most of Nancy's medical history was unremarkable, but there were a couple of items that drew my attention. She had suffered a broken arm after a fall while skiing two years before, and she'd had two automobile accidents in the last eighteen months. Nancy's family had a history of stroke and Alzheimer's disease. Her Braverman Nature Assessment identified her acetylcholine nature, and blood tests revealed a normal estrogen level, due to the Premarin (which we replaced with a natural bioidentical form of estrogen), but identified deficiencies in growth hormone and progesterone, testosterone, DHEA, and calcitonin (Miacalcin). Tests also uncovered osteopenia—the early stage of osteoporosis. While her original diagnosis of low hormone levels was accurate, there was no doubt in my mind that the majority of Nancy's complaints could be traced to her acetylcholine deficiency.

BALANCING YOUR
ACETYLCHOLINE NATURE

Acetylcholine deficiency can cause conditions such as memory lapses, trouble walking, and lethargy. Yet even these annoying problems are only early signs of the real trouble that may occur if you don't pay attention to brain chemistry. Now that you are aware of your nature, it is always best to treat relatively minor acetylcholine-based symptoms as early as possible.

Any acetylcholine deficiency can be corrected by using some combination of the seven treatment modalities: medications, hormones, supplements, diet, lifestyle, environment, and electrical treatments. The severity of your symptoms, however, will determine which type of treatment will work best for you. You can gauge the level of your deficiency by consulting your deficiency test score. A minor deficiency will range from 0 to 5, a moderate deficiency will range from 6 to 15, and anything over 15 is considered a major deficiency.

ACETYLCHOLINE-FRIENDLY
MEDICATIONS

Once you've balanced your acetylcholine by following the suggestions in the rest of this chapter, you should not need prescription medications. But until your acetylcholine is balanced, you may require some combination of prescription drugs. Pharmaceuticals designed to reverse a parietal-lobe acetylcholine deficiency work by affecting brain speed in some way. Talk to your doctor regarding drug choices and specific doses that are right for you. Dosage will vary significantly based on your height, weight, and gender. Each drug has specific properties that address a specific speed-related imbalance.

Bed-wetting (children) and adult patients with memory dysfunction: arginine vasopressin, or AVP

Memory enhancement for patients with minor memory loss: piracetam, vinpocetine (both of these are sold in specialty compounding pharmacies and on the Internet), galantamine (Reminyl)

Memory loss, Alzheimer's disease, and other dementias: donepezil (Aricept), rivastigmine (Exelon), neostigmine (Prostigmin), tacrine (Cognex), galantamine (Reminyl)

Muscle weakness and myasthenia: pyridostigmine (Mestinon)

Urinary disorders: bethanechol (Urecholine)

Vascular disorders: statin drugs

Visual disorders: pilocarpine (Salagen)

Many of the medications that Nancy's original doctor put her on were not appropriate for someone with an acetylcholine nature. I tapered her paroxetine (Paxil) for this reason (this drug addresses serotonin-related depression and can often be replaced by progesterone, growth hormone, or mood-enhancing supplements such as St. John's wort). Diethylpropion (Tenuate) was discontinued, as it addresses dopamine-related fatigue, and Nancy's lethargy wasn't related to dopamine—I could tell because her brain voltage was normal.

To my mind, none of the conditions related to Nancy's acetylcholine deficiency were at a point that would require pharmaceutical intervention. I took her off synthetic estrogen (Premarin) and switched her to a bioidentical estrogen, which has no negative side effects. Furthermore, bioidentical estrogen along with tyrosine and the herb rhodiola can have the same effect as weight loss drugs without the problematic side effects. My goal with Nancy—as it is with all of my patients—was to eliminate all drugs from her treatment program as soon as possible.

HORMONES

Hormones that augment acetylcholine are vital for health. Each of us loses different hormones at different rates, so we must monitor our hormone levels and supplement them as necessary. While the hormones listed at right are necessary for all of us, an acetylcholine nature will naturally use these more rapidly, and therefore require more supplementation. As with prescription medications, all issues related to hormone replacement must be resolved in conjunction with a medical doctor. Specific conditions, and the acetylcholine hormones related to them, include:

Appetite control: estrogen

Fluid retention: vasopressin

Kidney failure, anemia: erythropoietin

Lethargy: DHEA (dehydroepiandrosterone)

Memory loss, muscle loss: human growth hormone (HGH)

Metabolic disorders (weight gain): calcitonin (Miacalcin)

Osteoporosis: parathyroid hormone, estrogen, calcitonin (Miacalcin)

While Nancy's conditions did not require medications, they definitely called for hormones. She was given 18 mg. of natural growth hormone per month to address her memory, her metabolism, her muscles, and her bones. I also gave her 50 mg. per day of DHEA to restore her vigor, and 200 IU per day of calcitonin (Miacalcin) to stabilize her metabolism. Natural estrogen helped control her appetite and lose weight. Supplementing her estrogen was a good idea for her menopausal symptoms (dry vagina, low sex drive, and low mood) and for helping her control her appetite and lose weight, but using Premarin wasn't. I replaced that prescription with 0.5 mg. of estradiol—bioidentical estrogen—and combined it with 100 mg. of progesterone and a small amount (2.5 mg.) of testosterone, a combination known as PET. My clinical experience with thousands of women, as well as other clinical studies, has consistently shown that careful monitoring and supplementation of both male and female hormones when treating menopause symptoms achieves the most effective and longest-lasting results. Additional benefits of PET replacement therapy, particularly important in Nancy's case, include memory improvement from the estrogen, increased bone density from the progesterone, and improved vigor from the testosterone.

DIET

For many conditions—especially those present in the early stages of deficiency—you don't need a doctor's help to restore and maintain your acetylcholine balance. You can take matters into your own hands by following the nature-balancing suggestions for your diet and supplement regimen.

One of the easiest ways to keep your acetylcholine nature balanced is by making better food choices when you eat. When your acetylcholine is deficient, your body needs more of the nutrient choline, which begins as a B vitamin and is converted to acetylcholine. Choline is so important to cognitive function that food manufacturers are now adding it to a wide variety of products. The U.S. government has established that any food with 55 mg. or more of choline per serving can be touted as "a good source of choline."

Choline is a key building block needed to create myelin, the insulation surrounding the membrane of many neurons. Essentially, choline is a good fat that protects the body from potentially dangerous surges of electricity that course through it every day. In order for our brain speed to remain high, there needs to be enough insulation around the neurons so that information to and from the brain stays in the nerve fiber and does not dissipate as it passes from site to site. Studies report the value of choline in diseases such as Huntington's chorea, Alzheimer's, psychiatric disorders (particularly mania and mood swings), Tourette's syndrome, and ataxia (inability to control voluntary muscle movement).

Nature-specific diets are not about portion control or essential components. The important thing is to form a healthy habit of selecting acetylcholine-producing foods the majority of the time. When you do so, the occasional french fries and ice cream you sometimes crave will have little or no harmful effect.

The benefits of your acetylcholine diet will be evident after a few weeks as your body begins getting an adequate supply of choline to keep its acetylcholine flowing. Cognitive problems associated with memory and thinking will gradually improve. You can supplement your nature diet with any noncarbonated, nonalcoholic, sugar-free beverage you prefer. Round out a meal with any additional fruits and vegetables you like even if they don't appear in the acetylcholine list at right.

Choline is a natural component of plants and animal products. Foods highest in choline are egg yolk, meat, liver, and cereals. Unfortunately, often the best sources of choline are foods with high fat content, exactly the types of food people want to avoid when they are trying to lose weight. Consequently, when we diet, we may be unconsciously decreasing our choline intake, which is especially worrisome for those of us with an acetylcholine deficiency. Adult men require 550 mg. per day of choline, up to a maximum of 3.5 grams per day. For women, choline intake should be at least 425 mg. daily, with an upper limit of 3.5 grams. Foods that are high in choline include:

PER 6–8 OZ.

Almonds (100 mg.)	Liver, beef, cooked (840 mg.)
Artichokes, cooked (60 mg.)	Liver, chicken, cooked (600 mg.)
Beef, ground, lean, cooked (170 mg.)	Liver, turkey, cooked (440 mg.)
Broccoli, cooked (80 mg.)	Macadamia nuts (90 mg.)
Broccoli rabe, cooked, (60 mg.)	Oat bran (120 mg.)
Brussels sprouts, cooked (80 mg.)	Peanut butter (130 mg.)
	Pine nuts (100 mg.)
Cabbage, cooked (80 mg.)	Pork (180 mg.)
Egg, whole (500 mg.)	Shrimp, canned (160 mg.)
Egg, yolk (1.4 g.)	Soy protein powder (160 mg.)
Fish, cod, cooked (160 mg.)	Tomato paste (80 mg.)
salmon, cooked (130 mg.)	Wheat bran (150 mg.)
tilapia, cooked (160 mg.)	Wheat germ, toasted (300 mg.)
Hazelnuts (90 mg.)	

DEFICIENCY CRAVINGS

Just as people with a dopamine nature reach for sugar and caffeine for that extra burst of energy, if you have an acetylcholine nature, you probably crave fatty foods. Now you know why: because they deliver an instant choline boost. But too much fat circumvents the body's natural mechanism for production of acetylcholine.

TRIMMING THE FAT: CHOOSING
THE BEST SOURCES OF ACETYLCHOLINE

While it is important to eat foods high in choline, there are low-fat options available that work just as well as their high-fat counterparts.

HIGH-FAT CHOLINE FOODS	LOW-FAT CHOLINE FOODS
Avocado	Cucumber, zucchini, lettuce
Bacon	Canadian bacon
Bologna, frankfurters sausages	Lean chicken or turkey

HIGH-FAT CHOLINE FOODS	LOW-FAT CHOLINE FOODS (cont'd)
Cream	Skim milk
Egg fried in fat	Poached, boiled, or baked eggs
Fatty pork (spareribs)	Well-trimmed lean pork (ham)
High-fat cheeses	Low-fat cheeses
Ice cream	Ice milk, low-fat frozen yogurt
Liver	Fish
Nuts	Fruits and vegetables
Regular ground beef	Lean beef with all fat trimmed
Regular salad dressing	Reduced-calorie salad dressing
Sour cream	Low-fat yogurt, low-fat sour cream
Whole or condensed milk	Skim milk, buttermilk, nonfat powdered milk

ACETYLCHOLINE-BOOSTING DIET

If your acetylcholine nature has been diminishing, or if you are trying to enhance this biochemical as complementary to another nature, try this choline-rich diet. These menus span three days and can give you an idea of the foods you can eat that will increase your acetylcholine. How often you repeat this diet depends on your deficiency level. If you have a minor deficiency, follow the three-day course once a month; if you have a moderate deficiency, once a week. An extreme deficiency requires at least six days a week of this specific diet.

DAY 1

BREAKFAST	2 poached eggs with 2 teaspoons of caviar. 2 oz. celery salad with seasoned olive oil. 1 slice whole-wheat toast. Finish with a glass of grape juice.
LUNCH	6 oz. grilled chicken over cabbage salad with sage and raisins. Finish with an orange and a cup of green tea.
DINNER	8 oz. Caesar salad with 2 oz. cheese (skip croutons). 6 oz. horseradish-grilled salmon with 4 oz. couscous and 6 oz. broccoli. Finish with herbal tea.

DAY 2

BREAKFAST   8 oz. wheat germ cereal mixed with ¾ cup fresh, mixed berries, ⅓ cup mixed walnuts and almonds, with 1 cup skim or soy milk. Finish with ½ cup orange juice, freshly squeezed if possible, so as not to introduce preservatives or extra sugar.

LUNCH   8 oz. chicken soup with 1 slice whole-wheat toast. 8 oz. multicolored vegetable and tofu salad with olive oil and low-sodium soy sauce. Finish with water with lemon.

DINNER   Grilled vegetable mix with fava beans sprinkled with turmeric. 8 oz. beef or 8 oz. veal. Finish with low-calorie hot chocolate.

DAY 3

BREAKFAST   1 whole-wheat or wheat-free waffle with ½ tablespoon peanut butter and 2 oz. fresh berries. 1 soft-boiled egg dressed with 1 teaspoon olive oil and balsamic vinegar seasoned with cumin, garlic, pepper, and basil. Finish with a cup of coffee flavored with cinnamon.

LUNCH   4 oz. smoked salmon with 1 tablespoon low-fat cream cheese and lettuce, tomatoes, and onions on 1 slice whole-wheat bread. Finish with ½ cup grape juice.

DINNER   8 oz. lamb with 2 oz. mixed cranberries and almonds in 1 tablespoon olive oil and seasoned with rosemary. 4 oz. brown rice and 6 oz. steamed cauliflower and carrots. Finish with hazelnut herbal tea.

HEALTHY SNACKS   4 oz. steamed green soybeans (edamame); 1 slice tofu cheese; a boiled egg with 2 oz. carrots; 4 stalks celery with 2 tablespoons peanut butter; 2 oz. caviar on 1 slice whole-wheat or rye toast.

Our patient Nancy's thirty-five pounds of excess weight were the result of her low mood—she would eat to comfort herself—and her fat cravings. Substituting low-fat choline-rich foods at every meal eliminated her cravings and improved her mood.

VITAMINS AND SUPPLEMENTS

When we are healthy, we can get enough choline from the foods we eat. However, when the first symptoms of illness occur, this nutrient can be supplemented to avoid more serious symptoms, conditions, and medical treatments. Further, if you are sensitive to the loss of your edge or are looking to gain the Edge Effect, an easy fix is to keep up these nutrients through supplementation.

Readily available vitamins and supplements are an excellent way to ensure a steady supply of nutrients essential to the production of acetylcholine. Because they are brain-speed-oriented, they are best taken in the early morning through the afternoon to keep you sharp during the day: you don't want your brain racing at night, when it's time to slow down for proper rest. Absorption is best achieved when these supplements are taken half an hour before eating.

PHOSPHATIDYLSERINE

An impressive volume of research shows that phosphatidylserine, another modified amino acid, benefits acetylcholine deficiencies. We often recommend phosphatidylserine in our clinic when a patient is diagnosed with a memory disorder, early dementia, or depression. Multiple sclerosis patients may respond to phosphatidylserine as well.

ANTIOXIDANTS

Antioxidants are the ultimate brain food because they protect the membranes of brain cells by providing building blocks for those membranes. Antioxidants are common in many vegetables such as tomatoes, and many fruits, including blueberries, and can also be found in supplemental antioxidant formulas. Antioxidants are also thought to preserve membranes of brain cells by preventing oxidation of those membranes that would otherwise occur as we get older. (Free radicals are also associated with oxidation that damages cell membranes.)

I have developed a unique supplement formula, called Brain Memory, which you can readily reproduce. This formula contains GPC choline and phosphatidylcholine, two nutrients that imitate natural acetylcholine. It also includes huperzine-A (which preserves acetylcholine), N-acetyl-cysteine, and L-carnitine. L-carnitine is an amino acid thought to be helpful in lowering triglycerides, promoting weight loss, and building acetylcholine. N-acetyl-cysteine is an amino acid that helps detoxify many chemicals and is a strong antioxidant. This combination creates an acetylcholine precursor for myelin, which helps neurons process memory without losing speed. This formula will help to keep your edge fast and help decrease the symptoms of memory lapses, difficulty concentrating, confused thinking, and dry mouth.

Specific acetylcholine-related conditions are more responsive to certain supplements. The recommended daily allowance (RDA) is in parentheses.

Antioxidant that preserves acetylcholine: lipoic acid (100–400 mg.)

Attention deficit: deanol (100–200 mg.)

Memory problems: choline (men 550 mg., women 425 mg.), phosphatidylserine, glycerol phosphocholine (typically 1,000 mg.)

Metabolic disorders: conjugated linoleic acid (1,000 mg.)

Mineral that preserves acetylcholine: manganese (1–5 mg.)

Thinking problems: acetyl-carnitine, fish oils (up to 5 g.)

See the table on page 112 for suggested daily supplements and their recommended dosages.

LIFESTYLE

The acetylcholine nature is all about interactions with people, and a constant turnover of new ideas and activities. But your brain can't handle this constant barrage of new ideas forever without some preventive maintenance and biochemical replenishment.

Being alone once in a while is not punishment—it's a way to give

ACETYLCHOLINE BOOSTERS (SUGGESTED DAILY SUPPLEMENTAL DOSES)

	Minor Deficit (0–5)	Moderate Deficit (6–15)	Severe Deficit (15+)
Choline (GPC choline)	100 mg.	200 mg.	500 mg.
Phosphatidylcholine	500 mg.	1,000 mg.	2,000 mg.
Phosphatidylserine	50 mg.	100 mg.	200 mg.
Acetyl-L-carnitine	250 mg.	500 mg.	1,000 mg.
DHA (docosa-hexaenoic acid)	200 mg.	500 mg.	1,000 mg.
Thiamine	25 mg.	50 mg.	100 mg.
Pantothenic acid	25 mg.	50 mg.	100 mg.
Vitamin B_{12}	100 mcg.	200 mcg.	500 mcg.
Taurine	250 mg.	500 mg.	1,000 mg.
Huperzine-A	50 mcg.	100 mcg.	200 mcg.
Ginkgo biloba	50 mg.	75 mg.	100 mg.
Korean ginseng	100 mg.	200 mg.	500 mg.

your brain some time off to recharge itself. Try not to define everything you do in terms of whom you're with and what you're doing with them. This doesn't mean living as a hermit. It simply means making some time to be by yourself—reading a book, meditating, taking an extended walk, or praying—to provide resting time for your brain while it's awake. Try to allow for at least half an hour of solitary time every day.

If you don't enjoy reading, acetylcholine natures might find meditation quite remarkable. Meditation gives the mind a chance to relax and rejuvenate. Because you view the world through all of your senses, try the following visual meditation.

EXERCISE: VISUAL MEDITATION

Gaze at a photograph, drawing, inspirational image, or nature scene. Color, depth of field, and meaning are all important aspects in choosing an image. You can choose a photograph of loved ones, a postcard landscape or still life, or a personally signficant work of fine art. If you are looking at a picture of a religious object, you may find that it will help you create a spiritual connection. Whatever you choose, gaze at the image for a few moments, and then close your eyes and calmly try to re-create this image in your mind. Take your time. What makes this image important to you and why do you have a unique relationship with it? When you feel that you fully understand the image, open your eyes and see if your mental re-creation matches the actual object.

OTHER LIFESTYLE STRATEGIES

Someone with an acetylcholine nature relies on feelings and the ability to empathize with others. However, some decisions—health-related ones, for example—are better made based upon facts and logic. Rational people are not your adversaries—they just think differently than you do. And they provide balance for you. If you're unable to incorporate a little more logic and rationality into your nature, let others who possess these abilities lead the way once in a while. Either way, your brain again gets some time off to rest while awake.

Regardless of your nature, regular exercise is beneficial for muscle tone, strong bones, and good circulation. Although you may have the best of intentions, you seem to spend more time thinking about exercise than getting around to it. Studies have shown that aerobic exercise can restore acetylcholine, so it should become a regular part of your life. You'll need at least half an hour of aerobic exercise every other day. These activities include running, jogging, brisk walking, an aerobics class, bicycling, or anything else that increases your heart rate.

ENVIRONMENT

Your acetylcholine balance is particularly sensitive to the adverse effects of aluminum. Avoid aluminum cookware or utensils, and avoid products that may contain aluminum: baking powder, antacids, and water softeners. Aluminum can replace zinc in the neuron, and neurons without their zinc ions get tangled in their connections. If you don't read product labels, start now—your nature depends on it.

Violent films and TV, aggressive and foul language, and pornography are more than an affront to your sense of social decorum—they're a drain on your supply of acetylcholine. Your eyes are literally the entryway to the brain. The information they take in, both good and bad, affects your brain chemistry. For example, cognitive functions are damaged by violent visual stimuli. Your physical health is also at risk: watching violence increases your blood pressure and pulse and makes you more anxious. If you're more selective about your entertainment, you'll be choosing to preserve your nature.

As was the case with other pollutants such as PCBs, fertilizers, and pesticides, early warnings about electromagnetic fields (EMFs) were initially discounted. But studies have confirmed the hazards of concentrated exposure to magnetic fields and microwave radiation. Their negative effect on acetylcholine has been documented as well. So choose to live as far away as possible from power lines, stand away from and to the side of microwave ovens, use incandescent or full-spectrum lightbulbs instead of fluorescent ones, and always use the hands-free attachment for your cell phone. Studies show mixed results of fluorescent lights on ADD and of electromagnetic fields on mood, health, and obesity, but based on what I've seen in my office, these mixed results will later prove to have a direct effect on your nature.

No matter what your nature, you can create a restful environment by filling your personal spaces with soft lighting, gentle music, and pleasing scents. If you surround yourself with calm for at least a portion of every day, you'll accelerate the restoration of your acetylcholine balance.

GETTING INTO BALANCE

When your acetylcholine nature is unbalanced, your thought processes are immediately affected. You can't remember what you want to do, and you don't know what to do about that. You can't rally those closest to you, colleagues at work, or people in your community. You can't project what tomorrow will be, let alone next week or next year. You can't create a picture, a paragraph, an idea, a vision.

By following the steps described above, you can create a better balance by using all of the tools at your disposal to restore your acetylcholine. For Nancy, the path to better health didn't begin by dealing with her weight, her withdrawal from work and family, or her elevated cholesterol. The real solution to restoring Nancy's edge was a simple one: balancing her acetylcholine.

All of Nancy's conditions could be traced to diminished brain speed. When your brain speed begins to slow down, cognitive functions—memory, thinking, intuition, visual perception—are affected. Nancy's positive mood returned after a few nights of restful sleep and was reinforced by subsequent signs of progress. Her low levels of acetylcholine and associated hormones were the primary contributor to her complaints, and their replacement with natural alternatives was responsible for reversing her health decline. After two weeks her vigor returned, and she found herself diving into her caseload with renewed interest. Two weeks after that, her muscle and bone aches were gone, as were her memory lapses. She no longer had to work hard to remember details about her patients. With a lot less to worry about, and with her hormones properly balanced, Nancy had no trouble when it came to relations with her husband. Her trademark smile, absent for quite some time, returned.

After three months, once she had substituted low-fat versions of important choline-rich foods for the high-fat ones she was craving, Nancy had only ten more pounds to lose. She was back in the thick of things at work. Her thinking was clear, her intuition was intact, and her creativity was inspired. By reaching her Edge Effect, she was able to achieve her physical and mental peak. Her brain speed was optimized, and her Alzheimer's risk dropped significantly. Most exciting, she was able to regain her youthful brain energy and recover her old self—a size nine with balanced hormones, balanced acetylcholine, and a balanced life.

By following these suggestions, you too can balance your acetylcholine nature and restore yourself to full and abundant health.

ALZHEIMER'S DISEASE AND ACETYLCHOLINE

Alzheimer's disease is directly related to slowing down the activity of the brain, which is regulated by acetylcholine. The good news is that I've seen many cases of significant progress achieved, simply by following an acetylcholine protocol as outlined in this chapter. For example, I've treated a seventy-seven-year-old woman who could not tell me the date or the current president's name. After taking the entire program, including acetylcholine-friendly hormones and nutrients, she regained her entire memory and was able to address my staff by name. Another remarkable story involves a fifty-five-year-old salesman who came to me with the memory loss issues of a seventy-year-old man. Three years later his memory has been restored to that of a thirty-five-year-old. With Alzheimer's disease, as with any other condition affecting your mind and body, your health is in your hands. If you have any concern that you might be a candidate for this devastating disease, seek treatment as early as possible, using this book as your guide.

6

THE STABLE
GABA NATURE

IF YOU SCORED high on the Braverman Nature Assessment for GABA, then you are dominated by this neurotransmitter. The biochemical GABA (gamma-aminobutyric acid) has a calming, stabilizing effect on the brain. GABA prevents us from being too "juiced," too quick, and therefore ineffective.

In this chapter you will learn how to recognize your GABA nature and see how it affects all areas of your physical and mental health. More important, you will be able to identify as GABA-deficiency-related some of the specific ailments you might be experiencing, and learn how to correct a GABA deficiency. By addressing this deficiency, you will be taking both a step toward better health and a leap toward attaining the Edge Effect.

THE GABA NATURE
PERSONALITY PROFILE

The GABA nature is characterized by stability. Almost 50 percent of the world's population shares this nature, whose hallmarks are consistency, sociability, and concern for others. Luckily for the rest of us, GABA natures are the most dependable. If you have a GABA nature, you can be counted on to show up every day to do your job and to be there when others need you. When your GABA is in balance, your feathers remain unruffled when chaos swirls around you.

The ability to set goals, organize a project or activity, schedule, and administer, as well as such characteristics as punctuality, practicality, objectivity, levelheadedness, and confidence, all come naturally with a balanced GABA nature. Organization is paramount to you—at work, at home, in relating to others. Rigid schedules are your idea of heaven— they eliminate worry about uncertainty and ensure smooth sailing. Given these characteristics, GABA-dominant people naturally gravitate toward careers such as administrators, accountants, security officers, nurses, technicians, air-traffic controllers, news reporters, emergency medical technicians, meeting planners, bus drivers, and homemakers— the ultimate caretakers. No matter what the profession, the GABA-natured person is the one who tethers the group, who stays focused on the matter at hand, yet usually defers to the majority.

If you're GABA dominant, you're the consummate team player, on and off the field, and derive pleasure from fulfillment of every obligation and taking care of those you love. You're sensible, settled, not given to broad swings of emotions or outbursts of anger. Though you relish group activities, you cherish your one-to-one connections. Making others comfortable—both physically and emotionally—is the source of your own happiness. Marriage for you is a long-term haven. Keeping up with old friends is routine, as is the protection and nurturing of others, never more evident than within your own family. You're always available to advise, console, encourage, or just listen.

You probably believe in traditions and institutions, and relish your part in making them work, especially at a place of worship. You preserve conventions because they provide security for all. You look forward to group activities, especially holiday gatherings. Whether you are planning celebrations or networking events, these activities are more play than work. History books and biographies are on your reading list. Collecting memorabilia and creating scrapbooks for others to appreciate provides hours of entertainment. Tidying up is not a chore but a relaxing pleasure.

The Edge Effect for GABA occurs when you've maximized your GABA nature. These are the times when you feel you've had a strong nurturing effect on those around you. This might occur after you have hosted a holiday dinner for which you prepared everything from the turkey to homemade breads and desserts. You are satisfied that you have done a wonderful job, and your efforts are appreciated.

TOO MUCH GABA

It is possible to have too much of a good thing, as we've seen with the previous primary neurotransmitters. Producing too much GABA ratchets up your nurturing tendencies. At their worst, people with this personality expend their energy looking for love and opportunities to give care at the cost of being hurt when their own needs are not sufficiently met. Those with GABA natures rely heavily on their mates and authority figures for advice and can fall into the trap of continuously craving and following the judgments of their peers.

OUT OF BALANCE: GABA DEFICIENCY

But what happens—and how can you know—when your GABA starts running low? GABA is produced in the temporal lobes and is associated throughout the brain with calming, rhythmic theta brain waves. GABA is the major inhibitory neurotransmitter of the nervous system, which keeps all of the other biochemicals in check. GABA controls the brain's rhythm so that you function, both physically and mentally, at a steady pace. By regulating your internal rhythm, GABA directly affects your personality and determines how you handle life's stresses. When your rhythm is thrown off by a GABA deficiency, you may begin to feel anxious, nervous, or irritable.

A balanced brain creates and receives electricity in a smooth, even flow. When your brain is not producing enough GABA, your brain's electricity is generated in bursts. This is called a brain arrhythmia, or dysrhythmia, and it can upset your system in a variety of ways, none more pronounced than your emotional well-being.

The chart on the following page demonstrates a scale of conditions that can occur when your GABA is out of balance. The numbers on the left of the table correlate to the approximate number of brain arrhythmic events that occur during a half second of auditory and visual brain stress testing.

DEGREE OF DYSRHYTHMIA		GABA IMBALANCE
Mildly GABA deficient	1	Allergies, light-headedness, restlessness, transient muscle tension or aches
	2	Feelings of dread, blurred vision, protein cravings, impulsive attention errors, cold or clammy hands, butterflies in the stomach, feeling of a lump in the throat
	3	Dizziness, coughing or choking, temporomandibular joint syndrome, paresthesia (prickling or tingling sensation), phobias
	4	PMS, irritable bowel syndrome, night sweats, moderate to severe constipation/diarrhea
	5	Tachycardia (rapid heartbeat), mood swings, various mild pain syndromes, various anxiety disorders, hypertension
	6	Delusions, unexplained chronic pains, trigeminal neuralgia and other facial pains
	7	Short or violent temper, chronic insomnia, neuropathy (nerve pain), fibromyalgia (chronic muscle pain)
	8	Severe heart arrhythmias, carbohydrate cravings, severe migraines, rage
	9	Severe tinnitus, severe pain, manic depression, seizures
Severely GABA deficient	10	Marijuana abuse, alcoholism

GABA-RELATED ILLNESSES

For a GABA nature, or those with a GABA deficiency, the early warning signs of deteriorating health relate to loss of stability. Physically, you're pestered by annoyances from one part of your body after another.

Mentally, you start worrying about forgetting things that you never had to even think about before. This can show up in your body in a variety of ways and can affect any of the four major domains of brain function:

PHYSICAL ISSUES

Abnormal sense of smell—sensing abnormal odors

Action tremors

Allergies

Appetite or weight: significant change

Backache

Blurred vision

Butterflies in the stomach

Carbohydrate cravings

Cardiac arrhythmias

Chest pain or discomfort

Chronic pain

Cold or clammy hands

Constipation

Coughing or choking

Decreased libido

Diarrhea

Difficulty swallowing

Dizziness

Dribbling

Dry mouth

Excessive sleeping

Flushing

Headache

Hypertension

Hyperventilation

Hypotension

Insomnia

Instability

Irritable bowel syndrome

Lump in throat

Muscle loss

Muscle tension

Nausea

Night sweats

Paresthesia

Premenstrual syndrome or excessive menstrual bleeding

Protein cravings

Seizures

Shortness of breath

Slowness of physical movements

Stroke

Sweating

Tachycardia or palpitations

Tinnitus

Trembling, twitching, feeling shaky

Urinary frequency

Vomiting

PERSONALITY ISSUES

Adjustment disorders

Anxiety

Depression

Feeling of dread

Guilt or feelings of worthlessness/hopelessness

Lack of emotional maturity

Manic depression

PERSONALITY ISSUES (cont'd)

Mood disorders	Rage
Obsessive-compulsive disorder	Restlessness
Phobias or fears	Short temper
Poor emotional stability	Thoughts of death or suicide
Psychosis	

MEMORY ISSUES

Global memory problems	Poor verbal memory

ATTENTION ISSUES

Difficulty concentrating	Impulsive attention errors
Disorganized attention pattern associated with anxiety	(jumping the gun, erratic driving)
High anxiety	Inability to think clearly

With half of the population GABA-dominant, millions of people experience these symptoms every day. Tens of millions of symptom-specific prescriptions are written, but only a few address the GABA deficiency causing them. The value of *The Edge Effect* is in associating the earliest symptoms with a GABA deficiency and showing you what the easiest, least damaging, and most effective interventions are.

If you compare the above lists with those for the other natures, once again you will find symptoms and conditions that appear in more than one chapter. This repetition is caused by the fact that while there are four primary neurotransmitters, pairs often work in similar ways. For example, both dopamine and acetylcholine act as the electrical on switch for the brain: they create energy the body uses for power and speed. On the other hand, GABA and serotonin are the electrical off switches: they create electricity necessary for calming the body and promoting sleep. Because their functions are similar, similar symptoms may occur when either is deficient.

Also, the brain-mind-body connection has only a limited number of possible malfunctions. These malfunctions affect the rest of our system in similar ways. However, how a deficiency affects specific organs or systems varies by nature. For example, both GABA and acetylcholine deficiencies can cause frequent bowel movements, but for different reasons. Acetylcholine deficiencies affect metabolism, while GABA affects the rhythm of your intestinal tract.

GABA DOMINOES

Compared to some of the other nature deficiencies, GABA symptoms and illnesses are relatively minor. However, left unchecked, an unbalanced GABA nature, or a GABA deficiency in combination with a different nature, can be the first sign of health problems to come. The first metaphorical tile that falls during GABA dominoes is so subtle, you might not even think it is a problem. At the earliest point in low GABA production, you can't seem to shake a nagging headache. You're annoyed by constant burping every time you eat. Your sleep has been disturbed by night sweats once or twice. Soon you're experiencing occasional dizzy spells and clammy hands, and you can't remember what your best friend asked you to do for her today. And why are daily, routine tasks such a chore all of a sudden?

All of this would go away, you think, if you could just get a few nights of restful sleep. But that has become even more difficult now that you are experiencing muscle aches in your back and legs. Maybe a visit to a day spa, including a full-body massage, is the answer. It would at least give you a break from all those people who are starting to really annoy you with their neediness. Often you're jotting down reminders to yourself to do the things you always did without thinking about them. You find that much too frequently your day ends with much left undone, which makes the next day problematic. Those close to you may remark how you haven't been your usual self.

You decide to schedule a doctor's visit, especially since you've been experiencing shortness of breath and heart palpitations. At the doctor's office, you're relieved to hear that other than hypertension, which is causing the palpitations, you're not seriously ill. Your other symptoms can be attributed to stress, overwork, lack of sleep, and getting older. Your doctor recommends antacids and aspirin and tells you to spoil yourself for a change, instead of always taking care of others. She writes a prescription for beta-blockers for the elevated blood pressure, and one for a sleeping pill. You're not thrilled about having to take drugs, but you're confident that there's now something you can do to restore your usual orderly life.

And for a few months, things are normal. Then new problems crop up: cold hands and feet, persistent viral infections, weight gain, and depression that causes you to withdraw completely—from your work, from your community, from your family. Your conditions, albeit minor, are still real, as is their cause: GABA deficiency. The ultimate result of an untreated GABA imbalance is far worse. Without the proper medical attention, you could develop an immune system disorder and become susceptible to serious infections and diseases, ranging from Epstein-Barr syndrome to cancer. Your anxiety accelerates your pain, which leads to inflammation and eventually to premature aging. With all this worrying, you will grow old right before your eyes.

Although you might think this scenario is far-fetched, it is exactly what happens when a GABA deficiency is left unchecked. Consider Mary. When I first met her, I was perplexed as to why she was seeking treatment. Physically, she looked fine. However, she began telling me that although she looked neat and trim, the past five years had been rough. I felt for her as I looked at her strained face. A fifty-year-old school administrator who had spent her whole life helping others, she desperately needed help herself now. She was on the verge of tears as she described a litany of travails.

"I've been dealing with one condition after another. As soon as one complaint goes away, a new illness takes its place. My problems began a few months ago with a headache that was always with me. When over-the-counter remedies did nothing, I had my eyes checked and had a CAT scan of my head. Both were normal, but I still have a headache, which I'm learning to live with. I'm also living with burping, insomnia, tingling in my fingertips, asthma, chronic diarrhea, and palpitations. I've been married for twenty-five years, and for the first time my husband tells me that I'm snoring, and I'm not enjoying sexual relations as much as I used to. All these problems don't seem like much, but they're taking my mind off my job, my family, my friends. Everything is out of control. Now I am experiencing constant back and neck pain, but I'm afraid to have the surgeries the orthopedist is recommending. I feel like I'm falling apart, and I don't know where else to turn."

She went on to tell me that besides her physical complaints, she was totally befuddled about how to get anything done. Writing a grocery list was more than she could attempt. Where holidays once had been a time of excitement and joy, Mary now thought they came too frequently—and she dreaded them. She couldn't even attend parties or family gatherings others arranged, because she didn't want anyone to see her like this.

Mary's life, which had revolved around others, was becoming centered on the progression of her symptoms and her attempts to find cures. She was starting to feel guilty about concentrating so much on herself. She fretted that her issues would become burdensome to those who had always depended upon her. Fortunately, her children, at nineteen and twenty-five, were out of her home and starting lives of their own. But at work there were always students and their needs, and Mary felt that she was failing them every day.

Before she came to see me, Mary had visited a variety of other medical specialists. She was given an array of medications for her various complaints: albuterol (Proventil) for her asthma, beta-blockers for her palpitations, a seizure medication for her tingling, diphenoxylate and atropine (Lomotil) for her diarrhea, zolpidem (Ambien) for sleep, and oxycodone (OxyContin) for her back and neck pain. As for sex, her doctor scolded her when she brought up the subject, and told her that her other conditions were far more important to address. Another doctor actually told her that she had to make concessions in life, and enjoying sexual relations was one of them!

I did a complete workup on Mary, including taking her family history. Her family had a history of alcohol abuse, but Mary had managed to stay clear of that trap. She didn't have any traumatic childhood experiences, and she had experienced normal pregnancies, no sexually transmitted diseases, and no serious accidents. At five feet four inches and 104 pounds, she certainly wasn't overweight. Her diet was healthy, her cholesterol was normal, and she didn't smoke. In fact, other than a little experimentation with marijuana in her twenties, there wasn't anything remarkable at all in Mary's medical history. People like Mary—structured, organized, stable, consistent, punctual—would not likely have drastic deviations from norms when it came to their health background. It would have been a surprise if there had been something remarkable in her past.

Physically, Mary was in pretty good shape. She had lower-than-normal levels of progesterone, a female hormone, but she was on the verge of menopause, so low progesterone was not unusual for a woman her age. Her pulmonary function test came out normal, despite her asthmatic difficulty breathing. Her reproductive system was fine, so the answer to her sexual dysfunction was directly connected to her anxiety. Her bone density came back normal.

However, Mary's brain was far from healthy. Her Braverman Nature Assessment revealed the underlying cause of her complaints: a GABA deficiency and the rhythm disturbances that accompany it. Her physical symptoms were the direct result of her brain chemical imbalance. They could be summed up with one term: generalized anxiety disorder. The cause of her anxiety was decreased GABA production, which lets the nervous system run wild. When the nervous system's signals get crossed, the body responds with its own anxiety: we urinate too often, we produce too much gas, our hands become clammy, and the heart palpitates, among others. You may have noticed these conditions when you are feeling anxious about something.

Mary's constant anxiety was causing the rest of her physical problems. Simply put, her brain was sending the wrong signals to her organs. This was also the reason why there was no stability in Mary's life: no order, no job satisfaction, no sense of accomplishment, no certainty.

If Mary followed a conventional course, her condition would certainly have deteriorated, because conventional medicine never would have uncovered her GABA problem. With all of the drugs she was taking, side effects would be unavoidable. Amnesia could result from sleeping pills, addiction could result from painkillers, depression and a further loss of sex drive are common after taking beta-blockers, and constipation could result from taking Lomotil.

Mary, who had the highest regard for tradition, organization, and convention, was able to go against the grain for the sake of her own health. When we first met, Mary was concerned that my practice was too "alternative" compared to the rest of the medical establishment. However, when she discovered her nature and learned to restore it, she was able to open her mind to a new medical approach and restore the balance in her life.

BALANCING YOUR GABA NATURE

Any GABA deficiency can be corrected by using some combination of the seven treatment modalities: medications, hormones, supplements, diet, lifestyle, environment, and electronic aids. The severity of your symptoms will determine which type of treatment will work best for you. Gauge the level of your deficiency by consulting your deficiency test score. A minor deficiency score will range from 0 to 5, a moderate deficiency will score between 6 and 15, and a severe deficiency will go over 15.

GABA-FRIENDLY MEDICATIONS

Once you've balanced your GABA by following the suggestions in the rest of this chapter, you should not need serious medications. But until your GABA is balanced, you may require some combination of prescription drugs. The pharmaceuticals designed to reverse a temporal-lobe GABA deficiency work by affecting the systems that control the body's rhythm or stability. Each medication has specific properties that address a specific rhythm imbalance. Talk to your doctor regarding drug choices and specific doses that are right for you. Dosages will vary significantly based on your height, weight, and gender.

In the brain, there are about ten known GABA receptors. Because of this, there are a large number of GABA drugs available: each family targets a different type of receptor. Certain GABA drugs can treat a variety of illnesses. For example, Topamax, which was originally marketed as an antiseizure or manic depression medication, can be an effective medication for obesity, because GABA controls the anxiety related to overeating.

The following lists a range of conditions and the major GABA medications that treat them.

Anxiety: lorazepam (Ativan), alprazolam (Xanax)

Breast cancer and other forms of cancer: tamoxifen (Nolvadex)

Headache: phenytoin (Dilantin), divalproex sodium (Depakote)

Hypertension, cardiac arrhythmias: calcium channel blockers such as verapamil (Calan) and nifedipine (Procardia), and also betablockers

Insomnia: zolpidem (Ambien), clonazepam (Klonopin), temazepam (Restoril)

Manic depression: divalproex sodium (Depakote), carbamazepine (Tegretol), verapamil (Calcin)

Muscle pain: oxycodone (OxyContin)

Muscle spasm, nighttime twitches: clonazepam (Klonopin)

Muscle tension: diazepam (Valium), alprazolam (Xanax)

Neuropathic pain, diabetic pain, herpes pain, facial pain, leg pain: gabapentin (Neurontin), phenytoin (Dilantin), carbamazepine (Tegretol)

Obesity: topiramate (Topamax)

Panic attacks: alprazolam (Xanax)

Seizures: tiagabine (Gabitril), lamotrigine (Lamictal), primidone (Mysoline)

Sleep disorders: zolpidem (Ambien)

Stomach cramps (children): atropine and hyoscyamine, phenobarbital and scopolamine (Donnatal)

Tinnitus, dizziness, Meniere's: clonazepam (Klonopin), gabapentin (Neurontin), triamterene (Diazide), meclizine (Antivert), phenytoin (Dilantin), lamotrigine (Lamictal)

Other than the Ambien she was taking to sleep, the majority of the pills that Mary had been prescribed were intended to ameliorate symptoms, not to treat her GABA imbalance. My goal with Mary—as it is with all of my patients—was to eliminate all drugs from her treatment program as soon as possible. Once her GABA imbalance was fixed, Mary would not need any of these medications.

HORMONES

Each of the four primary neurotransmitters has a characteristic hormone associated with it. When a particular biochemical becomes deficient, a hormone comes in to take its place. Unfortunately, this only works for so long; it can't be sustained over time. The backup for GABA is endorphin, your own endogenous morphine. But when you use it up, you're in worse pain than you were before. At this point, many people who experience chronic pain might turn to marijuana, a drink, or an addictive narcotic. No small part of the OxyContin problem is people who crush the tablets, defeating the controlled-release mechanism. Others start taking it for pain but develop an addiction. Still others use it appropriately and wind up physically dependent but not addicted.

Each of us experiences a decline in different hormones at different rates and at different times in our lives, so we must monitor our hormone levels and supplement them—under a doctor's direction—as necessary. The GABA hormones are vital for everyone's health, whether you have a GABA deficiency or not. While the hormones listed below are necessary for all of us, a GABA nature will be more sensitive to their depletion and therefore require more supplementation. For example, progesterone deficiencies are linked to depression, diminished libido, weight gain, diabetes, osteoporosis, and immune system disorders. Other natural hormonal supplements that might be useful for a GABA deficiency include pregnenolone, which is a calming precursor of DHEA, and growth-hormone-releasing hormone (GHRH), which may shrink tumors and may enhance fertility.

DIET

For many conditions—especially those present in the early stages of a deficiency—you don't need a doctor to restore and maintain your GABA balance. You can balance your nature with nature-specific diet, vitamin, and supplement choices.

The easiest and most natural way to keep your GABA nature balanced is with diet. The goal of a GABA diet is to ensure that the body has enough raw materials—in this case complex carbohydrates—to create a steady supply of glutamine, the amino acid that is the precursor to GABA.

The more GABA-producing foods you eat, the more GABA you will be able to create. Following is a list of foods that are considered to encourage the production of GABA. If you can incorporate these into your diet, the occasional fast-food meal or sinful dessert will have no harmful effect at all. Add in as many different fruits and vegetables as you like to your

GABA diet, even if they don't appear in the list below. You can also have any noncarbonated, nonalcoholic, sugar-free beverage you prefer.

GLUTAMIC ACID/GLUTAMATE (FORMS GLUTAMINE) MGS. PER 6–8 OZ. SERVING

Almonds, tree nuts (10.3 g.)	Oats, whole grain (7.4 g.)
Banana (220 mg.)	Oranges, citrus fruits (210 mg.)
Beef liver (6.5 g.)	Potato (830 mg.)
Broccoli (740 mg.)	Rice bran (3.7 g.)
Brown rice (940 mg.)	Spinach (680 mg.)
Halibut (7.9 g.)	Walnuts, tree nuts (5.4 g.)
Lentils (2.8 g.)	Whole wheat, whole grain (8.6 g.)

DEFICIENCY CRAVINGS

Too many simple carbohydrates are bad for GABA-nature people—they calm the brain temporarily, but within one to three hours a GABA imbalance will begin again. GABA natures need to stay away from simple sugars, white flours, and wheat products in general, with the exception of whole grains.

GABA-BOOSTING DIET

If your GABA nature has been diminishing, or if you are trying to enhance this biochemical as complementary to another nature, try the diet found at right. These menus span three days and can give you an idea of the foods and quantities you can eat that will increase your GABA. How often you repeat this diet depends on your deficiency level. If you have a minor deficiency, then you should follow a three-day course once a month. If you have a moderate deficiency, you should follow a three-day course once a week. An extreme deficiency requires at least six days a week of this specific diet.

Important components of this diet are organ meats (especially liver), whole grains, vegetables, nuts, legumes, cantaloupe, oranges, and reishi mushrooms.

The benefits of your GABA diet will be evident after a few weeks as your body begins to get an adequate supply of glutamine to keep its GABA flowing. Daily anxiety symptoms such as headache and irritable bowel will dissipate. If you've been having trouble sleeping, you'll be amazed at how calm and relaxed you are at the end of the day. You'll fall asleep easily, sleep undisturbed, and awaken fully rested.

DAY 1

BREAKFAST ½ cup whole-grain cereal mixed with ½ cup bananas, ⅓ cup cantaloupe, ⅓ cup oranges, and ¼ cup almonds. Finish with raspberry herbal tea.

LUNCH 8 oz. grilled liver with 4 oz. multicolored vegetable salad with olive oil and vinegar and 1 slice whole-grain bread. Finish with citrus fruit salad and herbal tea.

DINNER 4–6 oz. grilled halibut with ginger. 1 medium baked potato topped with ½ teaspoon cinnamon. 6 oz. apple, raisin, and walnut salad with a splash of balsamic vinegar. Finish with a glass of rice milk.

DAY 2

BREAKFAST 4 oz. fruit mixed with 2 cups plain yogurt. Finish with 1 cup soy milk.

LUNCH 4–6 oz. lentil soup with 1 slice rye toast. Finish with a sliced banana with cinnamon.

DINNER 8 oz. grilled dark-meat fowl with ½ cup mixed portobello and reishi mushrooms. Finish with 6 oz. mixed berry smoothie.

DAY 3

BREAKFAST 6 oz. oatmeal sprinkled with raisins and caraway seeds. Lemon herbal tea.

LUNCH 6–8 oz. steamed or baked chicken breast cooked with 3 bay leaves. 6 oz. cauliflower, beet, and green bean salad mixed with olive oil. Finish with mango juice.

DINNER	8 oz. lean steak with 4 oz. jasmine rice and 6 oz. mixed grilled vegetable salad sprinkled with dill. Finish with banana puree and a touch of cocoa powder.
HEALTHY SNACKS	1 whole-grain nutrition bar; ¼ cup nuts; veggie burger on whole-wheat bun with tomato sauce and oregano; 4 oz. citrus fruit salad

VITAMINS AND SUPPLEMENTS

Even with the best of intentions, you might not be able to stick to your nature diet at all times. But your brain still needs its GABA. Readily available vitamins and supplements are an excellent means to ensure a steady supply of GABA nutrients. They are best taken from the late afternoon through the early evening—these supplements will help you relax, and you don't want to slow down in the morning, when you need to approach the day with vigor.

When we are healthy, we can get enough glutamine from the foods we eat. However, when the first symptoms of illness occur, glutamine and its complementary nutrients can be supplemented to avoid more serious symptoms, conditions, and medical treatments. Therefore, augmenting these nutrients becomes your first line of defense to regain wellness.

Inositol is a vitamin-like substance that is related to phosphatidyl-choline in that they work together to build and protect cell membranes. It is in the B complex family and produces a calming and relaxing effect by activating GABA and cyclic adenosine monophosphate. Inositol has been used to raise GABA levels, and the use of high doses (2 to12 grams per day) to relieve anxiety stemming from GABA deficiency is well established in psychiatry.

As with medications and hormones, specific GABA conditions are more responsive to certain supplements. For GABA natures, I have created a GABA-balancing program that I call Brain Calm. It contains valine, isoleucine, leucine, inositol, and the B complex vitamins. (In the body, inositol and glycerin, from the body's glucose, convert to a natural diazepam (Valium) that can calm the brain and keep you on an even keel.) This chemical is phosphotidyl and inositol, which has a GABA effect. This formula is the antidote for being edgy: it decreases the symptoms of anxiety, including trembling, hyperventilation, palpitations, ringing in the ears, and cold or clammy hands.

GABA BOOSTERS (SUGGESTED DAILY SUPPLEMENTAL DOSES)

	Minor Deficit (0–5)	Moderate Deficit (6–15)	Severe Deficit (15+)
Inositol	500 mg.	1,000 mg.	2,000 mg.
GABA (generally not well absorbed)	100 mg.	500 mg.	1,000 mg.
Glutamic acid	250 mg.	500 mg.	1,000 mg.
Melatonin	1 mg.	2 mg.	3–6 mg.
Thiamine	200 mg.	400 mg.	600 mg.
Niacinamide	25 mg.	100 mg.	500 mg.
Pyridoxine	5 mg.	10 mg.	50 mg.
Valerian root	100 mg.	200 mg.	500 mg.
Passionflower	200 mg.	500 mg.	1,000 mg.

Alternatively, you can take any of the following supplements alone for a specific ailment. The recommended daily allowance (RDA) for each is in parentheses, when available:

Anxiety: kava (none established)

Insomnia: inositol (none established)

Elevated blood pressure: taurine

Muscle spasms: branched-chain amino acids, including valine, isoleucine, and leucine (none established)

Muscle tension: B vitamins, especially thiamine (men 1.5 mg., women 1.1 mg.) or riboflavin (men 1.7 mg., women 1.3 mg.)

Psychosis: glycine

Seizures, pain, anxiety, insomnia: gabapentin (Neurontin) is essentially made from GABA and inositol

LIFESTYLE

If you have a GABA nature, you need to realize that your life doesn't have to be defined in terms of someone else. Doing something solely for your immediate enjoyment is healthy. In fact, you'll be much better at taking care of others once you learn to take care of yourself.

Regular aerobic exercise is of tremendous cardiovascular benefit—and it helps maintain your GABA. Exercise also works as a tranquilizer for people with a GABA nature by helping restore your GABA balance. So power-walk, jog, use a StairMaster or treadmill, or ride a bicycle for at least thirty minutes three times a week.

EXERCISE: GABA AEROBICS ROUTINE

This routine is great for any nature that requires aerobic activity: acetyl-choline, GABA, or serotonin. All you'll need is a pair of comfortable walking shoes, a watch, and a pair of handheld weights of no more than two pounds each.

The goal of this routine is to get you moving at a variety of paces. You will be walking around your home. If you can, walk outdoors, no matter what the weather. The fresh air can do wonders for your GABA.

Start off with a five-minute warm-up as you circle your home. Carry your light weights with you and pump your arms as you walk. Your pace should be one at which you can easily carry on a conversation.

For the next twenty minutes, pick up the pace. You want to reach the point at which you are panting but could carry on a brief conversation at the same time. Vary your terrain: walk up and down a staircase, or walk up and down a hill. Pump your arms faster as you go, bringing the weights to the level of your heart.

For the last five minutes, progressively slow down your pace. Take long strides and stretch your legs as you bring your walk to an end. Stop pumping your arms and carry the weights at your sides. Don't stop moving until you have walked a total of thirty minutes.

OTHER LIFESTYLE STRATEGIES

Someone with a GABA nature needs to take time out to pursue the health benefits of play. Everything you do does not have to be a means to an end. Try to think of a hobby or pastime you used to enjoy or always wanted to explore. Make the time to pick it up again or investigate it for the first time, and if you like the activity, incorporate it into your life.

As for relationships, remind yourself that they are a two-way street. You don't always have to be the giver—it's perfectly okay, and actually necessary, for you to be on the receiving end as well. Open yourself to help and comfort from others. Don't always be so quick to offer yourself—let others fend for themselves more often, and let them approach you for help first. Remember that GABA people risk their health when they can't say no to others at times. You'll never become a self-centered, me-first person, and you don't have to be—there are plenty of those people around. But you will be taking better care of yourself by allowing others in your life to take care of you.

Mary now power-walks regularly, which not only provides the aerobic benefit she needs but also lets her be alone so that she can concentrate on herself. She has learned to turn over meal preparation to her husband twice a week, and if he doesn't feel like cooking, they go out for dinner. Mary always wished that she could paint, and now she attends art classes once a week and makes time to paint. She lets the answering machine pick up some phone calls, and she's learned to say no once in a while when she would otherwise jump in to volunteer. All of these small changes make for big increases in Mary's overall GABA production.

ENVIRONMENT

Your GABA balance is particularly sensitive to the adverse affects of lead poisoning. Avoid contact with old paint and pipes, and read warning labels carefully when using paints, stains, and varnishes. Elevated lead levels are common in depressed people—as much as 10 percent of the American population. As added protection, wear a mask when working with toxic chemicals. The negative effects of chemicals in our environment disrupt the stability of the brain, making us edgy or nervous.

GETTING INTO BALANCE

As a GABA nature, you know when everything's right in your world because there's nothing remarkable about it: nothing stands out, nothing is out of place. There's a seamless transition from one activity to another, from one person to another, from one day to another. That's the rhythm of your balanced nature.

Unbalanced, there is discord everywhere: from substandard work to unfinished personal business and physical ailments in every part of your body. But now you know it doesn't have to stay that way. Now you know about the weapons at your disposal to restore your GABA and to regain your edge.

Nature-based treatment is not miraculous. It's just good medicine. Getting to the source of an illness by discovering your nature is the path to health. All of Mary's conditions could be traced to a rhythm disturbance in her brain—a GABA imbalance. And when your rhythm is disturbed, all of your brain waves are out of balance, all four pairs of lobes in the cerebrum are affected, and so all parts of the body start sending warning signals. It was no surprise that Mary's lungs, nerves, digestive system, and muscles all were screaming out to her. The real solution to Mary's myriad health problems was the natural one: balancing her GABA.

As I've said before, conventional medications are a vital part of restoring health but must be used judiciously. Mary was taking far too many drugs for her own good, and eliminating them was not only gratifying to Mary but especially pleasing to me. After two weeks of normal sleep, the tingling in her fingers disappeared, she was breathing normally, and her digestive system was back to normal. She no longer needed her seizure medication, albuterol (Proventil), or diphenoxylate (Lomotil). The beta-blockers for her palpitations, which were leading to depression, were also eliminated after two weeks. All of these were replaced by a single medication for generalized anxiety: alprazolam (Xanax). Her back and neck pains subsided gradually and disappeared totally after the first month. Then she said good-bye to her oxycodone (OxyContin).

GABA-natured people are ideal candidates for making small yet significant improvements. Because of their organization and administration skills, they are excellent at incorporating new routines into their lives and sticking to them. Mary was no exception. She switched to a GABA diet and supplements immediately. And she took the necessary steps to reduce stress, which only exacerbates anxiety. She was no longer a slave to every item on her daily schedule; she made sure to get to all of the important ones, and if a minor one was left undone, so be it. She learned to say no more often, and she made sure to allocate at least an hour every day for herself to read, walk in a park, window-shop, or simply take a long, restful bath.

After three months, Mary wasn't taking any medications—not even alprazolam (Xanax). Her edge was being totally addressed with her diet, supplements, and lifestyle. As a concession to her age, she continued to take progesterone to maintain a normal level. This helped her to maintain her GABA balance and to restore her sex drive.

That was a year ago. Today Mary is back to her former self: organized, consistent, stable, punctual, and capable. Mary's relationships with her husband and children markedly improved—she was able to provide the loving support to their lives that she longed to give. Mary can now forget about her five years of health travails. What she won't forget is her newfound knowledge about her nature. She knows now that maintaining the stability she holds in such high regard is all about maintaining her GABA balance.

By following these suggestions, you too can balance your GABA nature and restore yourself to full and abundant health.

7

—

THE PLAYFUL

SEROTONIN NATURE

THE BIOCHEMICAL SEROTONIN helps to resynchronize your brain so that every morning you begin with a fresh start. If you have a serotonin nature, you are among the 17 percent of the population who really know how to enjoy themselves. Associated with delta waves in your brain, serotonin affects your ability to rest, regenerate, and find serenity.

In this chapter you will learn about your serotonin nature and see how it affects all areas of your physical and mental health. More important, you will be able to recognize some of the specific serotonin-linked ailments you might be experiencing, and learn how to address a serotonin deficiency and attain the Edge Effect.

THE SEROTONIN NATURE
PERSONALITY PROFILE

If you have a serotonin nature, you know how to live in the moment. You are a realist, keenly responsive to sensory input, yet at the same time you can be impulsive. You love to participate in activities—whether at work or at play—for their inherent enjoyment, not as just a means to an end. You define achievement as getting something done immediately. You thrive on change: you'll alternate tasks and find new ways of doing repetitive ones, try new foods, pick up a new hobby, plan a different vacation every year. If you find yourself sticking to the same old thing, you'll shake things up just for the excitement of taking on a challenge—and overcoming it.

When balanced, a person with a serotonin nature is receptive to stimuli, in touch with both mind and body, often physically coordinated, and very resourceful. Your dominant neurotransmitter is serotonin, you're not put off by struggle, and you're undeterred by setbacks. If you don't consider work play, it's not worth doing. Your serotonin nature is ideal for professions requiring motor skills, hand-eye coordination, flexibility, and crisis management. Tools of every kind are considered extensions of the serotonin brain. Construction workers, oil riggers, truck and ambulance drivers, military personnel, hairstylists, bartenders, pilots, and computer programmers—who get to play with the most advanced and expensive tools—are all likely to have a serotonin nature. Professional athletes, movie stars, photographers, and fashion models would also likely owe their choice of a profession, and their ability, to their increased levels of serotonin. Serotonin dominance would also be essential for the troubleshooting business executive hired to save a floundering company; for surgeons, orthopedists, and chiropractors; for detectives and investigators; and for specialists in crisis intervention.

If there's excitement to be had, you're there. Parties and celebrations, computer and video games, casino gambling—all these are natural choices for you. Mountain climbing, hunting, target shooting, skydiving, hang gliding, skiing, and scuba diving all offer enough excitement to interest you. And you'll try just about anything as long as there's some element of excitement involved.

You are passionate in your relationships but refuse to be tied down. Equally important is that others recognize your freedom. You can be the life of the party, and others gravitate to you. You're optimistic, cheerful, and easygoing, and you can keep any conversation animated. You want everyone to join in and be part of your fun. You also have a special fondness for children, although a commitment to them can be overwhelming. You delight in playing with them, and if you don't have children of your own, being the favorite aunt or uncle comes naturally to you.

You're intensely loyal to coworkers, friends, and family. People appreciate your practical side and the way you make the best of any situation. Your friendships are many and varied, broad rather than deep.

Your impulsivity and desire for new experiences move you away from people before roots form. Your natural disdain for order and structure, along with your love of independence, can place a strain on your closest relationships.

The Edge Effect for a serotonin nature occurs when you've maximized your serotonin nature and can experience feelings of serenity throughout the day. These are the times when you experience the high that comes from taking part in activities others would find dangerous, including bungee jumping, motorboat racing, whitewater rafting, motorcycling, or just staying out all night carousing. When you play hard, your body is in serotonin overdrive, and you are having the time of your life.

TOO MUCH SEROTONIN

It is possible to have too much of a good thing. Producing too much serotonin can make you extremely nervous. You can become hesitant, distracted, vulnerable to any manner of criticism, and morbidly afraid of being disliked. In the extreme, someone with an excessive-serotonin personality is painfully shy and sees himself as inadequate and inferior. Such people are plagued by sadness, anger, and a desperate desire for interpersonal interaction, which, ironically, they are too fearful to attempt.

OUT OF BALANCE:
SEROTONIN DEFICIENCY

Produced within the occipital lobes, serotonin helps to create the electricity for sight and rest, and it also controls your cravings. The occipital lobes maintain your brain's overall balance, or synchrony, by regulating the output of all the primary brain waves. The four brain waves appear in varying combinations throughout the day, but at night serotonin allows the brain to recharge and rebalance. If these brain waves are out of sync, the left and right sides of your brain will be out of balance, and you might feel like you are going off the edge: you are overtired, out of control, and unable to get restful sleep.

When your serotonin is unbalanced, your brain's ability to recharge itself is compromised. Serotonin burnout can occur from experiencing too much excitement or not getting enough sleep. When this happen, you simply cannot think clearly. The following chart shows varying degrees of serotonin deficiency, measured by using EEGs or brain maps to track the number of synchrony abnormalities.

DEGREE OF DYSRHYTHMIA		SEROTONIN IMBALANCE
High serotonin	10	Perfect brain: complete left/right synchrony
	9	Constipation or irritable bowel syndrome, vaginal dryness
	8	Nausea, delayed sexual response, poor temperature regulation, blues
	7	Mild osteo-rheumatoid arthritis, mild hypertension, premature ejaculation, allergies, mild PMS, overexcitability or overemotionality, mild learning issues
	6	Insomnia, masochistic tendencies, conversion disorder, lack of coordination, dizzy spells, tinnitus, mild dysthymia (a disorder related to depression)
	5	Irregular heartbeat, obsessive-compulsive disorder, severe PMS, moderate dysthymia, shyness, persistent arthritis, uncontrolled hypertension
	4	Wide range of perimenopausal disturbances, loner behaviors, severe osteoarthritis, rheumatoid arthritis
	3	Addiction, bingeing, moderate learning disabilities, severe mood disorders and moderate depression
	2	Alcoholism, major depression, hypersomnia (sleeping for hours)
	1	No sleep for days, stroke, severe learning disability, schizoaffective disorder
Low serotonin	0	Prolonged severe drug experimentation, extensive hallucinogen use, thought confusion, schizophrenia

SEROTONIN-RELATED
SYMPTOMS AND CONDITIONS

For a serotonin nature, the early warning signs of deteriorating health are the result of a serotonin deficiency, which causes a disconnect between the mind and body. This disconnect can manifest itself in a variety of ways, including any of the following symptoms and conditions:

PHYSICAL ISSUES

Abnormal sense of smell
Abnormal sleep positions
Aches and soreness
Allergies
Arthritis
Backache
Blurred vision
Butterflies in stomach
Carbohydrate cravings
Choking sensation
Cold or clammy hands
Constipation
Diarrhea
Difficulty swallowing
Dizziness or light-headedness
Drug and alcohol addiction
Drug reactions
Dry mouth
Flushing or pallor
Hallucinations
Headache
High pain/pleasure threshold
Hypersensitivity

Hypersomnia
Hypertension
Insomnia and early-morning awakening
Lump in throat
Muscle tension
Nausea
Night sweats
Palpitations
Paresthesia
PMS or excessive menstrual bleeding
Premature ejaculation
Premature orgasm for women
Salt cravings
Shortness of breath
Tachycardia
Tinnitus
Tremor
Urinary frequency
Vomiting
Weight gain
Yawning

PERSONALITY ISSUES

Codependency
Depersonalization
Depression
Impulsiveness

Lack of artistic appreciation
Lack of common sense
Lack of pleasure
Loner behaviors

Masochistic tendencies	Phobias
Obsessive-compulsive disorder	Rage
Paranoia	Self-absorption
Perfectionism	Shyness

MEMORY ISSUES

Confusion	Too many ideas to manage
Memory loss	

ATTENTION ISSUES

Difficulty concentrating	Restlessness
Hypervigilance	Slow reaction time

Obviously, no one person will have all of these symptoms at once, and certainly some are more serious than others. The value of *The Edge Effect* is in associating the earliest symptoms with a serotonin deficiency and directing you toward the easiest, least damaging, and most effective interventions.

Once again, if you compare the above lists with those for the other natures, you will find that some symptoms and conditions appear more than once. This repetition is caused by the binary nature of the neurotransmitters. While there are four primary neurotransmitters, pairs often work in similar ways. For example, both dopamine and acetylcholine act as the electrical on switch for the brain: they create energy the body uses for power and speed. On the other hand, GABA and serotonin are the electrical off switches: they create electricity necessary for calming the body and producing sleep. Because their functions are similar, similar symptoms may occur when either is deficient.

Second, the brain-mind-body connection has only a limited number of possible malfunctions. These malfunctions affect the rest of our system in similar ways. However, how a deficiency affects specific organs or systems varies by nature. For example, deficiencies in both serotonin and GABA affect your ability to sleep. But too little serotonin can produce night sweats and the inability to sleep, while too little GABA will leave you feeling fatigued throughout the day.

SEROTONIN DOMINOES

An unbalanced serotonin nature, or a serotonin deficiency for a different nature, can set off a series of health problems. Serotonin dominoes might start with a loss of enthusiasm for your favorite activity, either at work or at home. For the first time in your life you have to give yourself a pep talk to enjoy yourself. Making the rounds of your associates and friends, entertaining them at lunch, meetings, or functions, takes effort. You don't enjoy your food, and you compensate for the lack of flavor with quantity. The result is that more than a few extra inches start to appear in unwanted places.

You're not enjoying your life very much—you figure you'd better get some more rest. But the deep, restful sleep that previously came so easily to you is now elusive at best. Some nights you don't sleep at all, which explains why you show up late, and unprepared, for work, which you never did before. When you are at work, you're not getting as much done. When your breath becomes labored and your chest begins to hurt, you decide it's time to see a doctor.

The doctor at first does not seem to be overly concerned. You're just one of his many patients afflicted by the modern world: working too much and playing too hard. He believes that your symptoms are all related to anxiety, and he gives you medication to combat it, along with sleeping pills. He reminds you to start taking care of yourself and lose some weight. He recommends a high-protein, low-carbohydrate diet.

Things begin to look brighter until your skin breaks out two months later for the first time in over fifteen years. When your synchrony is off, there's a disconnect between the right and left sides of your brain, between your mind and your body. In extreme cases, schizophrenia results—literally, a split represented by two distinct personalities. On the physical side, serotonin deficiencies can cascade into alcohol abuse or, worse, liver disease as you continue to self-medicate in your attempts to get yourself back on track.

Although you might think this scenario is far-fetched, it can happen when a serotonin deficiency is left unchecked. My patient Tom was a good example of this. When the thirty-five-year-old carpenter shuffled into my office, I saw immediately that at five feet ten inches and

210 pounds, he was considerably overweight. Tom sat there, visibly sweating in my climate-controlled office, and unburdened himself.

"Doc, I'm having some trouble. I can't sleep, and it's hard to breathe at times. I'm not getting enough done on the job. I figured I'd been working—and partying—too hard, and that must be it. And I know my weight hasn't helped. But I'm still young, I'm strong—I can deal with all that. But doc . . . I . . . um . . . I'm having trouble . . . in bed." He fidgeted before telling me, "I'm losing my erection after two minutes. Can it be time for Viagra already?"

Tom, like most people his age, took life for granted. He moved nonstop from work to socializing. He enjoyed everything he did in full measure. But for the past six months, things had been markedly different. His work wasn't up to par, and on the job he didn't feel like one of the boys anymore. He had to force himself to join his buddies after work in the local bar. When he did show up, he stayed on the periphery, drinking successive beers in virtual silence.

Weekends were mostly spent alone. He missed softball and basketball games because he wasn't motivated to play—and then felt guilty about letting his teammates down. He made excuses not to be with his girlfriend. His shortness of breath, excessive sweating, and insomnia, coupled with his withdrawal from his usual social contacts, concerned him enough to seek medical help.

The first doctor Tom saw had put him on a strict high-protein, low-carbohydrate diet, and Tom was diligent about everything he ate. He lost ten pounds in a month and a half. He slept okay when he took a pill, but he still didn't feel right. His sweating persisted, even when he was relaxing. He surprised himself by falling off a ladder at work. He broke up with his girlfriend when he was confronted with his sexual dysfunction. That's when he looked me up.

In my office, the Braverman Nature Assessment identified Tom's serotonin nature. And he did reveal one important concern: alcohol abuse. Tom was used to having three to four beers about five times a week, and binged at least once every week. Although he tried to maintain the diet his doctor recommended, he had fallen back into his old habits: loads of pasta, potatoes, fried foods. He ate virtually no vegetables, whole grains, or fish.

Tom's symptoms indicated a major disconnect between his mind and his body, which explained his physical symptoms, including his clumsiness. His withdrawal from everyone and everything was the sign of a descent into depression. By the time Tom came to see me, his serotonin levels were so low that his brain could no longer recharge itself and was burning out.

Fortunately for Tom, the party wasn't over. He found the source of his former, happier life: his serotonin nature. He had learned at a young age that there are things you can do—things you must do—if you are to keep the party going. Now he needed to replace bad habits with good ones that would increase his serotonin production effectively and safely.

BALANCING YOUR
SEROTONIN NATURE

Tom's excessive sweating, insomnia, and sexual dysfunction were worrisome enough. Yet these complaints were mere nuisances compared to the major ailments that were bound to show up if Tom didn't seek appropriate treatment. Early—and relatively minor—serotonin-based ailments can be directly treated with medications, hormonal means, alternatives such as diet and supplements, and lifestyle changes, including changes in the environment.

SEROTONIN-FRIENDLY
MEDICATIONS

Once you've balanced your serotonin by following the suggestions in the rest of this chapter, you should not need serious medications. But until your serotonin is balanced, you may require some combination of prescription drugs. These pharmaceuticals are designed to reverse an occipital-lobe serotonin deficiency by affecting the body's symmetry—its connection between the left brain and the right brain. Each of these medications has specific properties that address a specific symmetrical imbalance. For example, many serotonin medications actually reverse obsessive-compulsive behavior, which is the result of the brain being out of sync.

Any serotonin deficiency can be corrected by using some combination of the seven treatment modalities: medications, hormones, supplements, diet, lifestyle, environment, and electrical treatments. The severity of your symptoms, however, will determine which type of treatment will work best for you. You can gauge the level of your deficiency by consulting your deficiency test. A minor deficiency will range from 0 to 5, a moderate deficiency will range from 6 to 15, and a severe deficiency is considered anything over 15. Talk to your doctor regarding drug choices and specific doses that are right for you. Dosage will vary significantly based on your height, weight, and gender.

Following is a list of conditions related to serotonin deficiency and drugs that can be used to treat them.

Allergies: antidopamine agents such as diphenhydramine (Benadryl), cetirizine (Zyrtec), and loratadine (Claritin)

Anxiety: venlafaxine (Effexor)

Depression: paroxetine (Paxil), sertraline (Zoloft), citalopram (Celexa), fluoxetine (Prozac)

Dizziness or motion sickness: Dramamine

Insomnia: trazodone (Desyrel), nefazodone (Serzone)

Memory loss: Hydergine

Migraine headache: triptans

Nausea: ondansetron (Zofran)

Obsessive-compulsive disorder: clomipramine (Anafranil), fluvoxamine (Luvox)

Seizures: carbamazepine (Tegretol)

Sleep disorders and allergies: antihistamines

Medications can play a role in your recovery, but only if they are appropriate to your nature. Part of Tom's problem was that he was initially prescribed the wrong type of medication for a serotonin deficiency. I replaced his zolpidem (Ambien) and alprazolam (Xanax)—GABA-related medications for insomnia and anxiety—with trazodone (Desyrel) and paroxetine (Paxil), serotonin-related medications for insomnia and depression.

HORMONES

Each of us experiences a decline in hormone levels at different times in our lives and at different rates, so we must monitor our hormone levels and supplement them—under a doctor's direction—as necessary. While the hormones listed below are necessary for all of us, a serotonin nature will feel more out of sorts as the body naturally depletes them, and therefore will require more supplementation. For example, the hormone progesterone is vital for everyone's health, but especially if you are a serotonin type experiencing a deficiency. Progesterone deficiencies are linked to depression, diminished libido, weight gain, diabetes, osteoporosis, and immune system disorders, all of which are also serotonin issues. Natural hormones that can aid a serotonin deficiency include:

Adenosine: calms heart rhythm

HGH: improves sleep, encourages increase in bone density

Leptin: decreases appetite (not available to consumers yet)

Pregnenolone: increases total GABA levels

Progesterone (Prometrium): balances PMS, anxiety, insomnia

DIET

For many conditions—especially those present in the early stages of a deficiency—you don't need a doctor to restore and maintain your serotonin balance. You can restore your edge yourself with nature-specific diet, vitamin, and supplement choices.

The easiest and most natural way to keep your serotonin nature balanced is by making better food choices when you eat. The goal of a serotonin-balancing diet is to ensure that the body has enough tryptophan, an amino acid that can be converted to serotonin in the body. Tryptophan is found in many protein-rich foods, such as turkey, and naturally helps your body fall asleep. This is one of the reasons why you feel so satisfied, and tired, after a Thanksgiving meal. By ingesting enough tryptophan, you'll soon be able to discard any sleeping pill you've been taking.

Adults need about 200 mg. of tryptophan a day, though the body's need for tryptophan decreases with age. By eating foods high in tryptophan, it is easy to consume that amount. For example, there are 400 mg. of tryptophan in just one cup of wheat germ. A cup of low-fat cottage cheese contains 300 mg. of tryptophan, and a pound of chicken or turkey contains up to 600 mg.

The following is a list of foods that contain significant amounts of tryptophan. If you are trying to increase your serotonin levels, incorporate as many of these foods as possible into your diet each day. Be sure to round out a high-protein meal with lots of additional fruits and vegetables, even if they don't appear on the list below. You may also drink any noncarbonated, nonalcoholic, sugar-free beverage you prefer.

THE SEROTONIN DIET: TRYPTOPHAN FOODS

FOOD	AMOUNT	CONTENT (G)
Avocado	1	0.40
Cheese	1 oz.	0.09
Chicken	6–8 oz.	0.28
Chocolate	1 cup	0.11
Cottage cheese	1 cup	0.40
Duck	6–8 oz.	0.40
Egg	1	0.40
Granola	1 cup	0.20
Luncheon meat	6–8 oz.	0.50
Oat flakes	1 cup	0.20
Pork	6–8 oz.	1.00
Ricotta	1 cup	0.30
Sausage meat	6–8 oz.	0.30
Turkey	6–8 oz.	0.37
Wheat germ	1 cup	0.40
Whole milk	1 cup	0.11
Wild game	6–8 oz.	1.15
Yogurt	1 cup	0.05

DEFICIENCY CRAVINGS

Those with serotonin natures, especially where there is a deficit, will crave simple carbohydrates such as pastas and rice, as well as salt, all of which promote the release of stored serotonin, producing the expected serenity high. However, too much sodium is extremely bad for the body, especially if you have high blood pressure, and too many simple carbohydrates will lead directly to weight gain. Salt, salty snacks, and simple carbohydrates should be avoided.

An equally important issue for serotonin natures is limiting alcoholic beverages. While they can be tempting and definitely help you keep your edge, their long-run effects can be devastating. Limiting your alcohol intake to two drinks per day no more than twice a week will keep you satisfied without damaging your brain and body.

SEROTONIN-BOOSTING DIET

If your serotonin nature has been diminishing, or if you are trying to enhance this biochemical as complementary to another nature, try this diet. These menus span three days and can give you an idea of the foods you can eat that will increase your serotonin. How often you repeat this diet depends on your deficiency level. If you have a minor deficiency, then you should follow a three-day course once a month. If you have a moderate deficiency, you should follow this once a week. An extreme deficiency requires at least six days a week of this specific diet.

The main components of this diet are protein foods high in tryptophan, as well as complex carbohydrates.

DAY 1

BREAKFAST	6 oz. cream of wheat or rice cereal mixed with 2 oz. fresh fruits and 1 cup whole milk.
LUNCH	4 oz. egg salad with paprika and scallions, tomatoes, and lettuce on 2 slices of rye bread. Finish with iced tea.
DINNER	8 oz. Greek salad prepared with olive oil sprinkled with marjoram. 8 oz. ground turkey with whole-wheat pasta in tomato sauce sprinkled with 1 oz. cheese. Finish with black cherry tea.

DAY 2

BREAKFAST   2 eggs, scrambled, with seasonings such as turmeric, garlic, pepper, cumin, and tarragon with 1 nitrate-free sausage. Finish with ½ cup freshly squeezed orange juice.

LUNCH   4 oz. roast turkey with 4 oz. avocado-mint salad with tomatoes and black olives, dressed with safflower oil and sesame seeds. Finish with a cup of mocha.

DINNER   4 oz. mackerel cooked with basil and thyme with 4 oz. salad of corn plus red and black beans. Finish with 8 oz. vegetable juice sprinkled with Tabasco sauce.

DAY 3

BREAKFAST   Wheat germ sprinkled on 4 oz. multicolored apples and almonds and ½ cup cottage cheese. Finish with chamomile tea with lemon.

LUNCH   4 oz. lean pork cooked with mustard seed and black pepper. 5 oz. cucumber salad mixed with red pepper, lemon peel, chervil, 1 oz. blue cheese, a touch of olive oil, and 2 tablespoons balsamic vinegar. Finish with sugar-free lemonade.

DINNER   Broiled dark-meat chicken cooked with rosemary and garlic. 8 oz. brown rice seasoned with cayenne pepper. 6 oz. multicolored broiled vegetable salad, including asparagus, tomatoes, carrots, onions. Use the drippings from the chicken with added savory as your salad dressing. Finish with a cup of instant chocolate drink and ½ cup of berries.

HEALTHY SNACKS   2 oz. cheese with grapes; 1 cup of plain yogurt; 4 oz. egg salad on rye toast; granola bar; 1 baked sweet potato; 1 small bran muffin; 1 cup of raw string beans sprinkled with marjoram.

ALLERGIES: LOW-HISTAMINE DIET AND LOW-SEROTONIN DIET

Serotonin deficiencies often occur as allergies. There is some evidence that a diet that eliminates additives and foods high in histamines may lessen the severity of allergic reactions. If you have allergies or have experienced symptoms related to allergies, including sneezing, congestion, and watery eyes, you might want to consider the following lists of permitted foods and of foods to avoid.

PERMITTED

Beverages: fresh milk, tea, homemade fruit juice, mineral water

---

Cereals: freshly baked breads and cereals (not packaged)

Condiments: salt, pepper; other condiments to be taken only as
    dried leaves; vinegar only if label indicates no additives

---

Fats: butter, olive oil

Fruits: any in moderate quantities (many contain natural salicylates)

Meats: fresh meat, eggs, and fish only, in small quantities
    (no luncheon meats)

Sweets: homemade only, without additives

Vegetables: any in fresh state except beans, spinach, and cabbage
    (including sauerkraut); tomatoes permitted in moderation

AVOID

Food items likely to have additives: colored beverages, wines and
    other alcoholic beverages, artificial sweeteners, luncheon meats,
    ice cream, many yogurts, and ready-made, commercially
    available desserts

Other items: colored toothpaste, colored cosmetics

VITAMINS AND SUPPLEMENTS

Even with the best of intentions, you might not always be able to stick to your nature diet. But your brain still needs its serotonin. Readily available vitamins and supplements are an excellent means to ensure a steady supply of serotonin nutrients. Serotonin-boosting supplements are best taken from the late evening up until bedtime, as they are made to help put you to sleep.

These serotonin-related natural substances can work as effectively as many medications, although not as quickly. For example, tryptophan supplements have been shown to have a positive effect on everyday problems such as carbohydrate cravings, low blood sugar, aggressive behavior, and insomnia. Available by prescription, tryptophan is also a mild, natural growth hormone stimulator. In more extreme cases, suicidal patients, as well as agitated, depressed ones, do well with tryptophan supplements. A combination of tryptophan at night and tyrosine in the morning often mimics the effects of many antidepressants. Tryptophan is also beneficial in some forms of schizophrenia, in Parkinson's, and may even help with progressive myoclonic epilepsy.

I have developed a unique serotonin supplement formula, called Brain Mood. This formula contains thiamine, niacinamide, folic acid, vitamin B$_{12}$, pantothenic acid, 5-hydroxytryptophan, and St. John's wort. Niacin is the best-studied vitamin for reducing cholesterol, but a variant called niacinamide is also used for mood stabilization and treatment of depression and alcoholism. This formula promotes brain-mind-body connectedness and balance among the four main brain rhythms: beta, alpha, theta, and delta. It is helpful for decreasing the symptoms of insomnia, sleep disorders, backache, headache, shortness of breath, PMS, and phobias. Adequate Brain Mood can get you the Edge Effect: a cascade of wellness, serenity, and physical health.

As with medications and hormones, specific serotonin conditions are more responsive to certain supplements, listed below. The recommended daily allowance (RDA) for each is in parentheses, if known.

Attention deficit, sleep disorders, and concentration problems:
5-hydroxytryptophan (100–500 mg.)

Breast cancer: melatonin (100–200 mg.)

Constipation: magnesium (400–1,000 mg.)

Depression: tryptophan (500–2,000 mg.), St. John's wort (none established)

Difficulty metabolizing tryptophan: B$_6$ (100–500 mg.)

Insomnia: melatonin (1–3 mg. before age forty; older patients can take up to 6 mg.)

Low mood or blues: fish oils (none established), zinc

Weight loss and appetite control: hydroxycitric acid (250–1,500 mg.)

SEROTONIN BOOSTERS (SUGGESTED DAILY SUPPLEMENTAL DOSES)

	Minor Deficit (0–5)	Moderate Deficit (6–15)	Severe Deficit (15+)
Calcium	500 mg.	750 mg.	1,000 mg.
Fish oils	500 mg.	1,000 mg.	2,000 mg.
5-HTP	100 mg.	200 mg.	400 mg.
Magnesium	200 mg.	400 mg.	600 mg.
Melatonin	⅓ mg.	½–2 mg.	1–6 mg.
Passionflower	200 mg.	500 mg.	1,000 mg.
Pyridoxine	5 mg.	10 mg.	50 mg.
SAM-e	50 mg.	100 mg.	200 mg.
St. John's wort	200 mg.	400 mg.	600 mg.
Tryptophan	500 mg.	1,000 mg.	1,500–2,000 mg.
Zinc	15 mg.	30 mg.	45 mg.

To support his serotonin, so that we could eventually take him off trazodone (Desyrel), we started Tom on melatonin supplements. We later added St. John's wort and fish oils, which would, in time, replace the paroxetine (Paxil).

LIFESTYLE

A serotonin-nature diet with supplements is part of a healthy lifestyle that can tether you so you don't completely drift away. Additionally, be sure to include regular aerobic exercise. Exercise is important for the serotonin nature because it resets the brain just as sleep does. Use the exercise in the GABA chapter as a starting point. Because serotonin natures enjoy physical activity, try different ways to modify the exercise to changes things around for you. Make sure that no matter what type of aerobic activity you pick, you keep it up for at least thirty minutes three times a week. If you need to be around people in order to motivate you to exercise, join a gym.

The risk of the serotonin nature is that while you're so focused on enjoying yourself today, you don't consider how you will feel tomorrow. So while you don't have to become something you're not, a squirrel saving acorns for winter, you do have to learn that you can't do everything you want all of the time! You'll never be in danger of becoming a hermit. But let someone else be the life of the party once in a while, so you'll be around—in mind and body—to enjoy all the parties.

A serotonin nature can always stand a little introspection. Adding spirituality to your activity-laden days—whether in the form of prayer, meditation, yoga, or chanting—would establish your connection to something other than yourself. A feeling of peace and calm allows your brain some time to rest, to restore itself while awake.

EXERCISE: MEDITATION THROUGH CHANTING

A chanting exercise is great for a serotonin nature: it shuts your thinking pattern off, blocks negative thoughts, and slows the mind and body down in order to resynchronize. With a chanting meditation, you can get all of the advantages of sleeping while you are awake. The following exercise is a simple rhythmic chant. Follow the directions until you know this chant by heart. Then feel free to play around with your own internal message.

Lie on the floor in a room with a comfortable temperature. Don't lie in bed or relax on the couch: you are not supposed to fall asleep! Set a timer for five minutes and relax.

Close your eyes. Inhale through your nose as much air as your lungs can hold. Hold for a count of two, and then forcefully release all of the air in your lungs. Repeat for a total of five deep breaths.

Clear your mind of all extraneous thoughts. With your eyes still closed, say the following phrase aloud: "Life is the sum of its parts. I deserve to be healthy and happy." Repeat the phrase slowly, over and over, following the same cadence, until the timer rings.

Open your eyes. Again inhale through your nose as much air as your lungs can hold. Hold for a count of two, and then forcefully release all of the air in your lungs. Repeat for a total of five deep breaths.

ENVIRONMENT

Your serotonin balance is particularly sensitive to the adverse effects of PCBs, pesticides, and certain chemicals found in plastics, because the neuron damage caused by exposure to these hazards can make you unable to rest. Rinse all of your food, especially fruit, thoroughly. Be observant about pesticide spraying if you live near or visit farms. Never go near burning plastics. As for PCBs, be cognizant of where your fish comes from, opting for wild fish whenever possible, and drink water only from reputable bottlers or after it has been filtered. Bearing in mind warnings about mercury in fish, try to avoid the following: Atlantic halibut, king mackerel, Gulf Coast oysters, pike, sea bass, shark, swordfish, tilefish (golden snapper), and tuna (steaks and canned albacore).

GETTING INTO BALANCE

Anticipating everything you do with excitement, and deriving enjoyment in the doing, is a marvelous approach to life. Sensing what's in front of you, and coordinating your body to respond in the moment, is the key to your serotonin nature. With the tools now at your disposal, you're free to restore your edge.

All of Tom's conditions could be traced to the disturbed symmetry in his brain—a serotonin imbalance. It would take some time to get Tom's weight back to normal, but he didn't have to wait long to feel better. I adjusted his medication at his initial office visit, and within days he was able to sleep peacefully. Treating his depression quickly took the edge off his nervousness. His breathing returned to normal, and his excessive sweating disappeared within two weeks.

Within a month, Tom didn't have to tell his friends he was feeling better—they could see for themselves when he started dropping by again to tell a few jokes and share a laugh. After two months, all of the elements of Tom's treatment program were contributing to regaining his serotonin balance, and he was able to stop taking the trazodone (Desyrel) and paroxetine (Paxil).

Tom's dietary discipline has returned dividends, too—conscientiously staying away from simple carbohydrates and alcoholic beverages, he lost forty pounds and looks great. He's popular once again with his associates and friends. He's got a new girlfriend—and he's actually looking forward to a steady and deepening relationship. He has no reason to think about sexual dysfunction anymore: he's got staying power and control over his ejaculations.

Tom understands that life isn't an unending party. But he can enjoy every day as long as he listens to his body when it tells him his brain needs adjustment. And now he knows how to balance his serotonin without getting himself into trouble.

By following these suggestions, you too can balance your serotonin nature, and restore yourself to full and abundant health.

PART III

BALANCING YOUR BRAIN IN SICKNESS AND HEALTH

8

—

THE BRAVERMAN

PRESCRIPTION

Now THAT YOU have identified your nature and your deficiencies, you can begin to take control of your total health. In the previous sections you learned how your brain works and how to identify your nature and your deficiencies, and you were introduced to a variety of techniques and treatments that can build up a biochemical deficiency or maintain your nature. In this section you will learn how to deal with specific illnesses or symptoms you may be experiencing, both in the brain and in the body. In this way you can control your health now and create abundant health for your future by reaching the full Edge Effect.

The good news is that life expectancy is on the rise. The population's average age is rising, and now there are more senior citizens than ever before. A child born in 1997 can expect to live at least 76.5 years, 29 years longer than a child born in 1900. A man who reaches age sixty-five in 2004 can expect to live an additional 15.8 years, and a woman can expect to live an additional 17.6 years.

The goal for all of us then becomes learning how to take control of our aging process so that we can enjoy lasting health. Healthy aging is associated with an increased degree of brain function. To achieve this, we must learn how to balance and enhance our brain.

This chapter outlines what I call the Braverman Prescription. This prescription contains all of the information you need to be able to take control of the aging process right now and to achieve lasting health. It includes a general understanding of how your body ages, a simple eating plan that anyone can follow, and detailed instructions on how to enhance brain function. By understanding your true nature and following these three simple guidelines, you can halt premature aging and fully enjoy the rest of your life.

Whether or not you are currently experiencing symptoms, the path to total health should begin with a complete physical with a board-certified doctor. You can be a proactive part of your treatment by informing your physician about the results of your Braverman Nature Assessment. Let your doctor know about your nature and your biochemical deficiencies, and work with him or her to put together a treatment program that is best for you.

THE PAUSE MODEL
OF AGING AND DISEASE

There's no way around it—you begin aging the moment you're born, and the process doesn't stop until you die. But the problems we associate with aging are in large part the result of declines in our body's production of hormones as we grow older, and the problems that these cause for our body's electrical signals and the four main neurotransmitters, dopamine, GABA, acetylcholine, and serotonin. When hormone levels get too low, aging accelerates, and your body can function as though it's far older than your chronological age. If you're deficient in acetylcholine, you lose brain speed and your brain ages faster than the rest of your body. You might be only sixty-five, but you could experience loss of memory that would be comparable to that of a ninety-year-old.

I refer to these hormonal changes as *pauses*. The concept of pauses is based on the idea of menopause, the hormonal changes faced by every aging woman. Because hormones regulate all of the systems in the body, this experience can be related to all organs and systems of both men and women.

If a doctor knows a patient's biochemical nature and is able to identify which particular pause a patient is experiencing—which primary neurotransmitter there's a deficit in—she can treat symptoms and illnesses most efficiently. Furthermore, with this information, a doctor can estimate the rate at which a patient's system is aging and determine what needs to be addressed in order to slow down the process.

New studies suggest that the brain can be taught to reignite these hormone systems and actually resurrect your aging body. I have seen this countless times in my office. For example, a thirty-year-old man came in with the beginning stages of andropause, commonly referred to as male menopause. His symptoms included fatigue and a decreased libido, both of which most men do not experience until they are in their seventies. By balancing his acetylcholine nature with growth hormone and a nature diet, we lowered his cholesterol, and his testosterone actually increased! By following our plan, this man was able to delay the progression of andropause, and his life returned to a more normal, age-appropriate state.

The body undergoes various pauses from head to toe. Many of them parallel emotional changes, the most typical being a "mid-life crisis." By age fifty, most individuals have gone through at least one, if not several pauses. Even by age forty, partial pauses can have significant impact on an individual's well-being, energy, and total health. Fortunately, hormonal levels are easy to assess with simple blood tests. Be sure to ask your doctor for the appropriate tests based on your age.

PAUSE	DECLINE	TYPICAL AGE OF ONSET
Electropause	Electrical activity of brain waves	45
Biopause	Neurotransmitters	Dopamine: 30 Acetylcholine: 40 GABA: 50 Serotonin: 60
Pineal pause	Melatonin	20
Pituitary pause	Hormone feedback loops	30
Sensory pause	Touch, hearing, vision, and smell sensitivity	20–40
Psychopause	Personality health and mood	30
Thyropause	Calcitonin and thyroid hormone	50
Parathyropause	Parathyroid hormone	50

PAUSE	DECLINE	TYPICAL AGE OF ONSET
Thymopause	Glandular size and immune system	13/puberty
Cardiopause/ vasculopause	Blood flow, increase in blood pressure	40
Pulmonopause	Lung elasticity and function with increase in pulmonary pressure	50
Adrenopause	DHEA	30–60
Nephropause	Erythropoietin	40
Somatopause	Growth hormone	30–50
Gastropause	Nutrient absorption	40
Pancreopause	Blood sugar level	40
Insulopause	Glucose tolerance	40
Andropause	Testosterone in men	40–50
Menopause	Estrogen, progesterone, and testosterone in women	30–55
Osteopause	Bone density	30
Dermopause	Collagen, vitamin D synthesis	35
Onchopause	Fingernails, toenails	40
Uropause	Bladder control	45
Genopause	DNA	40

THE PAUSES AND STRESS

A person whose pauses begin sooner than they should is probably under great stress. Such a person might end up with dermopause at thirty, while others who are less stressed will not begin this pause until age fifty. In high-stress regions in United States, such as New York City, a greater number of men die at sixty-five than is the case in Hawaii, where the average male lives to the age of seventy-seven.

When brain stress is high, hormonal imbalances start very early on. Pauses progress more quickly, and imbalances feed each other as total health breaks down. We slide downhill faster and faster, especially if our brain isn't in good shape to begin with. For example, I have met with women in their thirties who are already experiencing perimenopause, the series of changes that culminates in menopause. Changes in progesterone make them cranky and moody and increase the severity of PMS. Imbalances in their estrogen/progesterone ratio cause early hypertension and panic disorders and eventually will lead to cardiac problems.

DELAYING THE PAUSES

By jump-starting the brain into health through medication, hormonal and vitamin supplements, diet, and exercise, we can cause our body's hormonal levels to rise, delaying the aging process. While you can't stop a genetically programmed pause, such as menopause, by increasing your body's production of estrogen, you may be able to delay it a year or two, or possibly more, and you can certainly prevent it from occurring too early.

In the discussions that follow, you will learn which of the four major neurotransmitters is involved in each of the pauses and what you can do to balance your body and delay onset of the pause. The earlier you begin to deal with hormone loss, the better results you are going to get.

For treatment instructions, please refer to the chapters in Part II that discuss each of these biochemicals in detail. If your symptoms are mild, you can begin by altering your diet or lifestyle by incorporating the various biochemical programs. If your symptoms are more than moderate, read through the information pertaining to various medications and hormone treatments, and then seek help from a physician.

PAUSES OF THE BRAIN

ELECTROPAUSE

Electropause is the change in brain chemistry that affects brain function. Electropause is influenced by changes in the brain's voltage, speed, rhythm, and synchrony. Symptoms include loss of memory, loss of emotional balance, depression, anxiety, personality disorders, mood swings, and in extreme cases psychosis. I divide these losses into the four biochemical categories: decreases in brain voltage can be directly related to dopamine, decreases in brain speed are related to acetylcholine, decreases in brain rhythm are related to GABA, and an unsynchronized brain is related to serotonin.

CONDITION	BRAIN AGE	BIOLOGICAL AGE
Alzheimer's	120	60
Parkinson's	95	70
Attention deficit disorder	50	7

VOLTAGE	RESULTING CONDITION
10 percent decrease	Blues
30 percent decrease	Obesity
70 percent decrease	Addiction
90 percent decrease	Schizophrenia/dementia

BIOPAUSE

Brain aging and deterioration—measured by losses in the brain's voltage, speed, rhythm, and synchrony—regulate all of the other pauses. Biopause is responsible for the cascade of all the other pauses and their related illnesses and symptoms. In terms of your total health, biopause is probably the most important pause to delay. By balancing the levels of all of your neurotransmitters, you will be able to put off the biopause and increase your chances of long-term health. As an added benefit, when you enhance your levels of these same neurotransmitters enough to delay biopause, you'll also achieve the Edge Effect.

PITUITARY PAUSE

The pituitary pause affects the pituitary gland and hypothalamus. The secretion of growth hormone declines between the ages of thirty and fifty, causing muscles to shrink and fat to increase. Other symptoms include anorexia, compulsive water drinking, sleep rhythm reversal, rage behavior, hallucinations, and obesity. Keeping the brain youthful and more energetic by boosting acetylcholine and dopamine might contribute to slowing this genetically programmed hormonal loss.

SENSORY PAUSE

Sensory pause affects all five of your senses. Hearing begins to decline between the ages of twenty and forty and worsens faster in men than in women. The loss of hearing impairs cognition as well as your overall mental health. Nutrients such as zinc and niacin can help, and certainly keeping the brain young by boosting your acetylcholine and dopamine is recommended. Your sense of smell declines slowly beginning around the age of forty, and more rapidly after sixty-five. Since olfactory cells are actually part of the brain tissue, a deficiency in any of the primary biochemicals, especially acetylcholine, may lead to this problem. Increased difficulty seeing nearby objects begins in the forties. Ability to see fine details does not deteriorate until the seventies. The loss of vision impairs cognition as well as your overall mental health. Nutrients, particularly antioxidants, have been shown to slow a variety of sight disorders. Acetylcholine and dopamine are most significant for sight health.

PSYCHOPAUSE

Worldwide studies of older adults have documented a 15 to 25 percent prevalence of serious mental disorders that first occur later in life. Organic mental disorders such as Alzheimer's disease and related dementias affect approximately 10 percent of persons older than sixty and as many as 50 percent of those older than eighty-five. While neuropsychiatric conditions can occur at any age, the elderly have particularly high rates of alcohol and substance abuse, dysthymia and depression, anxiety, schizophrenia, and personality disorders.

Decreased cognition results from decreased acetylcholine. An increase in the blues occurs due to decreased dopamine and serotonin. Overall personality disorders worsen if there is a decrease in GABA production. Anxiety increases when there is decreased GABA, when synchrony is reduced from the loss of ability to manage sleep cycles. The symptoms listed on the next page are signs of psychopause. If you are experiencing any of these, see a doctor immediately.

PHYSICAL SYMPTOMS OF PSYCHOPAUSE

Abnormal sense of smell

Allergies to peanuts, walnuts, or bananas

Autonomic hyperactivity

Backache, headache

Butterflies in the stomach

Chest pain or discomfort

Cold or clammy hands

Coughing, choking

Diarrhea

Difficulty swallowing

Dizziness or light-headedness

Dry mouth

Fatigue

Flushing and pallor

Muscle tension, aches, or soreness

Numbness or tingling

Sexual dysfunction

Shortness of breath, hyperventilation

Sleep disorders

Sweating

Tachycardia, palpitations

Trembling, twitching, feeling shaky

Urinary dribbling, incomplete bladder emptying

PSYCHOLOGICAL SYMPTOMS OF PSYCHOPAUSE

Decreased libido

Depersonalization or derealization

Difficulty concentrating

Fear of people or social events

Feeling of dread

Hypervigilance

Rage, extreme temper

Restlessness

SIGNS AND SYMPTOMS OF DYSTHYMIA (LOW MOOD) OR DEPRESSION

Cognitive problems (difficulty paying attention, memory disturbance)

Decreased desire for food or sex

Decreased involvement in usual activities

Decreased physical activity (psychomotor retardation)

Difficulty getting through routine tasks

Increased physical activity (psychomotor agitation)

Insomnia, early-morning awakening, or oversleeping

Loss of vigor or energy

Self-destructive thoughts

SIGNS AND SYMPTOMS OF DEMENTIA

Failure to recognize and identify familiar objects despite intact sensory function

Impaired attention and overall decline in processing speed

Impaired judgment

Impairment in abstract thinking

Language problems (aphasia)

Motor skill problems despite physical capacity

Significant impairment of short-term and long-term memory

PAUSES OF THE BODY

THYROPAUSE

The thyroid gland synthesizes the hormones thyroxine (T4) and tri-iodothyronine (T3), iodine-containing amino acids that regulate the body's metabolic rate. Adequate levels of thyroid hormones are necessary in infants for normal development of the central nervous system, in children for normal skeletal growth and maturation, and in adults for normal function of multiple organ and systems. Thyroid hormones increase the activity of membrane-bound enzymes, increase heat production, and stimulate oxygen consumption. Thyroid hormones also affect tissue growth and maturation, help regulate lipid metabolism, and increase intestinal absorption of carbohydrates. Thyroid hormones and dopamine have similar chemical structures, and influence one another.

SIGNS AND SYMPTOMS OF HYPOTHYROIDISM

Ankle edema

Cold, dry, thick, scaling skin; dry, coarse, brittle hair; dry, longitudinally ridged nails

Cold intolerance

Constipation

Diminished food intake or weight gain

Diminished libido

Generalized muscle weakness; delayed relaxation of deep tendon reflexes

Lethargy, decreased vigor

Mental clouding, depression

Normal or faint cardiac pulse; indistinct heart sounds; cardiac enlargement

Round puffy face, slow speech; hoarseness

Slow thinking

THYMOPAUSE

Beginning at puberty, your immune response declines slowly. Serotonin regulates the immune system, and serotonin agents can boost immunity, but an excess of serotonin can trigger arthritis. Dopamine agents also regulate the immune system but can consequently suppress auto-immune reactions.

CARDIOPAUSE

After age forty, many people experience up to a 20 percent decline in maximum heart rate during exercise because the heart becomes less responsive to dopamine and estrogen stimulation from the nervous system. Surprisingly, symptoms can include memory loss and anxiety. Cardiopause can be controlled via exercise, diet, and maintaining a youthful and less anxious GABA brain. By building up all of your natures and sleeping adequately, you are less likely to make wrong choices about behaviors that are destructive to the heart.

VASCULOPAUSE

Vasculopause affects your blood vessels and usually occurs around age forty. As the diameter of vessels narrows and the arterial walls stiffen, there can be a 20 to 25 percent increase in systolic blood pressure. Anxiety and a deficit of GABA are particularly destructive to blood vessels, because during a state of anxiety, your blood vessels will tense up. Getting adequate rest is a significant treatment, as is boosting your serotonin levels so that you can relax. All of the brain's biochemicals can ultimately impact blood flow throughout the entire body. Increased dopamine and aerobic exercise can strengthen the vascular system; increased acetylcholine keeps blood vessels flexible.

PULMONOPAUSE

Starting at the age of fifty, and definitely by seventy, most of us will lose up to 40 percent of our maximum breathing capacity. Pulmonary function is a strong predictor of overall longevity. Anxiety, stress, and exposure to various chemicals in the air contribute greatly to the deterioration of the lungs. Building up all of your biochemicals, particularly GABA, will have a great impact on lung longevity. Aerobic exercises can also help develop greater lung capacity.

ADRENOPAUSE

Between the ages of thirty and sixty, the adrenal glands' secretion of DHEA—which slows the growth of cancers and boosts immunity—declines. After age seventy, production of the stress hormone cortisol soars. Symptoms can include changes in memory and attention, depression, lack of energy, loss of libido, irritability, anxiety, panic attacks, paranoia, and increased appetite. Supplementation of hormones and nutrients and even hydroxycortisone may help. Although this pause is genetically programmed, building up the brain maintains the entire hormonal and nutritional component of the body. The adrenal gland is supplemental tissue to the brain's dopamine and adrenaline, and therefore it is less likely to kick in and burn out if your dopamine is kept high.

SOMATOPAUSE

Twenty to 40 percent of muscle mass can be lost by the age of ninety, especially if you do not exercise. Symptoms can include loss of memory, mental faculty, and muscle strength. Routine exercise is the best way to prevent most muscle loss. Growth hormone and amino acids may be beneficial. While boosting all the brain's biochemicals can help, dopamine is the most stimulating to muscle growth. GABA reduces tension, so when you are balanced your muscles don't hurt. Acetylcholine keeps your muscles from drying out.

MENOPAUSE (MALE AND FEMALE)

The first hormonal changes that lead to menopause can occur in women as early as thirty-five, and these can last ten to fifteen years. For women over the age of fifty, there is a dramatic decline in production of progesterone and testosterone. Estrogen starts to decrease earlier, around the age of thirty. What's astonishing to me is that I am seeing bone density loss in so many patients as young as eighteen. Other symptoms include loss of memory and other cognitive deterioration, as well as hair thinning and loss. Early supplementation with natural hormones and vitamins that boost GABA and dopamine might diminish the negative impact on the bones, the brain, and the hormones it produces. Male menopause, or andropause, typically *begins* in men between forty and fifty. Male menopause progresses slowly, over thirty years as testosterone supplements are increased.

OSTEOPAUSE

Bones begin to weaken after age thirty, which can lead to osteoporosis, especially in women. Hormones, calcium, and other nutrients may help. Although this is primarily a hormonal problem, the younger the brain and body are, the better the absorption of nutrients and hormones that are used to treat this. Therefore, boosting your acetylcholine and dopamine levels becomes critical to osteopause treatment, as long as the boost in these two biochemicals does not make you feel too edgy.

DERMOPAUSE

Changes in collagen and connective tissues cause skin to lose elasticity in later years. The rate at which skin ages is frequently genetic, relating to its ability to retain moisture. Yet the younger your brain is, the less your whole body dries out. Since the brain dehydrates with age, boosting dopamine and acetylcholine is very important—after all, acetylcholine is the moisturizer for the entire body. Topical medications such as Retin-A and maintaining a healthy diet can also help.

KEEPING THE PAUSES
FROM CONTROLLING YOUR BRAIN

As you can see, keeping your brain young and vibrant delays the onset of these pauses and hence slows down the aging process. Conversely, experiencing any of the pauses can throw your brain off, because an unhealthy body can wear down the brain. For example, the metabolic slowdown experienced in thyropause can actually decrease further dopamine production. By controlling the health of your body you can better protect your brain.

Virtually any physical disease or pause may produce anxiety and brain rhythm disturbances that wear out the brain. For example, andropause or any other pause accelerates electropause. When the brain burns out during biopause, the whole cycle of pauses begins.

Another example involves our immune system. When immunopause begins, the entire immune system slows down. As this occurs, osteoarthritis and joint wear and tear become more likely. Attempts to strengthen your joints with growth hormone and glucosamine are critical because a brain that is constantly in pain from arthritis or even minor joint problems wears itself out.

Toxic metals accelerate all pauses—this remains a very serious problem in our society. Heavy metals such as lead and cadmium are toxic to the brain and body and exist in many forms. For example, I often see individuals with elevated lead levels despite the fact that lead has been removed from gasoline and paint. Elevated lead levels are often found in psychiatric syndromes such as bulimia, psychosis, depression, and lupus. Elevated cadmium levels are common in smokers or people who live around smokers, and contribute to high blood pressure. Also, elevated copper levels contribute to depression. Elevated mercury levels may occur in some individuals who have problems with dental fillings. Aluminum has been implicated in memory loss.

THE RAINBOW DIET

One of the simplest ways to maintain your neurotransmitters, and subsequently slow down the pauses, is through your diet. In the nature chapters, there were specific diets recommended for boosting each of the biochemicals. The basic nature diet strategy to remember is that dopamine is boosted by a high-protein diet with fruit sugars; eggs, caviar, sardines, fish oils, and olive oil all raise acetylcholine. GABA is increased with vegetables, and serotonin is boosted by poultry and complex carbohydrates.

If you want to boost all of your biochemicals and achieve total health, you need to follow a program that incorporates all the nature-specific diet recommendations and adds essential nutrients as well. I advise my patients to follow what I call the Rainbow Diet. This diet will help you lose weight, lower your blood pressure, and improve your cholesterol profile. You will feel young, energetic, and—most important of all—healthy.

The Rainbow Diet incorporates all the different colors of the rainbow—red, orange, yellow, green, blue, indigo, and violet—into the meals we eat. Foods with a variety of colors have different nutrients, and no one supplement is equal to all the great nutrients you can get from fresh foods. These foods—fruits, vegetables, proteins, and complex carbohydrates—can be used in order to achieve your optimal weight results and improve your overall health.

As you know, the rainbow has seven colors, but it does not have any white! On the Rainbow Diet, "white" foods are avoided. These include white flour and foods made from it, such as bread and pasta; white rice; butter and margarine; and salt and refined sugar. White flour, white

---

CRITERIA OF THE RAINBOW DIET

Very high in vegetables of all colors, 4–6 servings a day
High in fruits of all colors, 4–6 servings a day
Multicolored spices 3 times a day
Multiflavored herbal teas 3 times a day
Very high in fiber-rich whole grains
Low in saturated fat and cholesterol
Low in trans fats
Low in sodium
Low in refined grains
Low in unhealthy oils
Low in sugar-rich foods and beverages
Moderate in low-fat proteins, 2 servings a day

---

rice, and sugar are bad choices because they don't have much nutritional value and also have a high glycemic index, which means that during digestion they break down quickly into simple sugars and are easily stored as body fat. These foods increase your risk for heart disease, constipation, obesity, and even some cancers. Butter and margarine are both harmful to cardiovascular health—butter because of its saturated fat, and margarine because of the trans fats it contains. And of course we all consume too much salt.

GOALS FOR THE RAINBOW DIET

At each meal, try to eat 80 percent fruits, vegetables, and grains and 20 percent protein food. Your protein should be fish as much as possible, but can also include chicken, turkey, and beans. Stay away from red meat and fried foods. Eat garlic, as it promotes healthy blood flow. Avoid caffeinated beverages, especially if you have high blood pressure. Take a multivitamin with minerals, antioxidants (especially vitamin C, vitamin E, and zinc), linoleic acid, and coenzyme Q_{10}.

Eat less saturated fat to avoid cholesterol problems. Saturated fats are found in many foods, including fatty meat, whole milk, most cheeses, ice cream, butter, lard, coconut oil, and palm oil. These foods directly contribute to increasing your cholesterol more than anything else you eat. Eating less fat will also help you eat fewer calories and keep your weight down. Losing extra weight can lower your cholesterol, too. Choose low-fat or fat-free cheeses, sour cream, and yogurt. The fats you do eat should be healthy ones—olive oil is an excellent choice, as it contains monounsaturated fatty acids, which are proven to lower cholesterol and improve overall lipid profile.

Use herbs, salsa, and spices instead of rich sauces, gravies, and extra salt. Bake, broil, boil, or steam foods. If you cook with fat or oil, use just a little or, better yet, none at all. Try nonstick pans and cooking spray. Trim the fat from meat before cooking.

Choose foods high in fiber such as fresh vegetables and fruits, which level off blood sugar. Do not skimp on protein and fat to make room for larger amounts of carbohydrates. Protein and fat give the body energy, help balance blood sugar, and keep cravings at bay. If you eat sweets on an empty stomach, you'll experience blood sugar surges followed by lows that trigger the desire for more sweets or carbohydrates.

TIPS FOR HEALTHY EATING

First and foremost, do not overeat. Use a measuring cup, measuring spoons, or a food scale to find out how much you are eating and what your serving sizes are. Write down what you eat and how much you eat. If it looks like too much, it probably is. Most people are surprised by how much they eat once they weigh or measure out their meals.

Another good tip is to always eat to lose weight, even if you don't think you should be dieting. If you weigh more than is recommended, your body stores fat, which may cause your cholesterol to increase; this can start a whole cascade of problems. Cut calories by eating smaller amounts of food. Do not skip meals; just eat a little bit less. Eat more slowly; take time to taste and enjoy your food. Help your pancreas to work better by keeping your blood sugar stable—frequent meals help maintain a balance of pancreatic hormones necessary for consistent and ongoing fat release.

Your body gets hungry every three to five hours. Impulse bingeing is usually a result of poor planning. If you eat at regular times every day and without going too long between meals, you will be less likely to overindulge. So always have three meals a day with two healthy snacks in between. People who snack between meals find it easier to lose weight because they actually take in fewer calories during their three main meals. Typically, bad snack foods are low in nutrients, high in sugar, high in fat, or contain refined carbohydrates, inhibiting the optimal fat loss environment. Even healthy snacks such as fruits can, when eaten by themselves, spike blood sugar and insulin levels. So rather than a muffin, which is full of sugar and refined white flour, consider a piece of whole-grain bread with one slice of turkey breast, a tomato slice, and spinach. Walnuts and almonds are a good snack choice in small quantities.

Supplement your diet with an antioxidant formula. A quality formula contains vitamin C, vitamin E, zinc, and other substances that neutralize free radicals, which can cause cellular damage if left uncontrolled. Lastly, make sure to get enough sleep. When the body and mind are well rested, cravings for carbohydrates often vanish.

RAINBOW DIET SAMPLE MENUS

Here are sample menus with many choices for each meal. You can mix and match any breakfast with any lunch and any dinner. Always have a drink with your meal. Try freshly squeezed orange or grapefruit juice, caffeine-free green tea, herbal tea, skim or soy milk, or water or no-salt seltzer with lemon. Use sugar substitutes if necessary.

BREAKFAST

Choice 1: 1 or 2 soft-boiled or poached eggs with olive oil, balsamic vinegar, and a pinch of cayenne pepper

Choice 2: Fat-free plain yogurt with berries and walnuts, almonds, or pumpkin seeds

Choice 3: Omelet with some cut-up vegetables sprinkled with turmeric (made in a nonstick pan)

Choice 4: Bran oatmeal with nuts, berries, and unsweetened soy milk

Choice 5: Pink grapefruit (sweeten with sugar substitute), 1 poached egg, and fresh spinach leaves

Choice 6: Caesar salad with 1 boiled egg, spinach, celery, carrots, and 4 oz. fresh turkey or chicken dusted with paprika

Choice 7: ½ cup cantaloupe, 1 slice whole-wheat toast with 1 tablespoon almond butter, 1 cup nonfat yogurt

Choice 8: ¼ cup egg whites scrambled with ½ cup veggies, 2 tablespoons olive oil, and a pinch of cumin, with 1 slice whole-wheat toast

Choice 9: ¾ cup bran flakes with ½ cup skim milk and ½ cup berries, 1 whole-wheat English muffin

Choice 10: 1 small whole-wheat bagel or 1 whole-wheat English muffin with 1 tablespoon low-fat cream cheese, dusted with allspice

Choice 11: 1 multigrain waffle or 2 whole-wheat waffles with ½ cup raspberries

Choice 12: 1 multigrain waffle or 2 whole-wheat waffles with ½ cup mixed berries

Choice 13: 1 slice whole-wheat toast with olive oil and seasonings

Choice 14: 1 cup bran flakes with 1 cup skim milk and 1 cup berries

Choice 15: 1 cup berries, 2-egg omelet with ½ cup vegetables, seasoned with fresh sage

LUNCH

Choice 1: 4–6 oz. warm sardines with 1 tablespoon pesto or olive oil with balsamic vinegar and seasonings, 2 cups multicolored lettuce salad with garlic safflower oil dressing

Choice 2: Tuna (mixed with olive oil, balsamic vinegar, and coriander) on whole-wheat bread

Choice 3: Rainbow salad—lots of different-colored vegetables with 1 hard-boiled egg and 1 slice low-fat cheese, dressed with olive oil, balsamic vinegar, parsley, and thyme

Choice 4: Piece of baked chicken, spinach salad dressed with 2 tablespoons olive oil, basil, dill, and a splash of vinegar

Choice 5: 6 oz. salmon with herbs, 1 cup salad dressed with olive oil and lemon juice

Choice 6: 1 bowl chicken soup made with whole-wheat pasta, seasoned with rosemary

Choice 7: 2 cups yogurt mixed with handful of nuts, berries, and other low-glycemic-index fruits

Choice 8: Turkey, chicken, or fish served with steamed vegetables, seasoned with freshly grated ginger

Choice 9: 1 cup vegetable soup, sandwich of 1 slice low-fat cheese, 2 slices tomato, and mustard on 2 slices whole-wheat caraway-seeded bread

Choice 10: 1½ cups spinach salad with 3 oz. skinless chicken breast, seasoned with marjoram, 1 tablespoon olive oil, and 1 tablespoon vinegar

Choice 11: 2 slices turkey breast, ¼ cup sprouts, 3 slices tomato, and mustard on whole-wheat pita, ¼ cup apricots

Choice 12: 1 cup salad with 1½ cup garbanzo beans, 1 cup yellow corn, 1 oz. walnuts, 2 tablespoons olive oil, and 1 tablespoon vinegar

Choice 13: 2 slices turkey or beef, 1 slice low-fat cheese, lettuce, 3 slices tomatoes, mustard on 2 slices whole-wheat bread, 1 piece fruit

Choice 14: 2 oz. water-packed tuna, 2 slices tomato, 2 leaves lettuce, and 2 tablespoons mustard on 2 slices whole-grain bread, 1 orange

Choice 15: ¾ cup hummus, red and green pepper strips, and 5 whole-wheat sesame crackers for dipping

DINNER

Always accompany dinner with a fresh salad with olive oil and balsamic vinegar. If you have to eat late, keep it light—for example, turkey, chicken, fish, tofu, or beans with salad or soup with vegetables or chicken soup with 1 slice whole-wheat bread.

Choice 1: Grilled chicken (6–8 oz.) with fresh basil, with ½ cup brown rice, 1 cup grilled vegetables, bananas with cinnamon or cocoa powder for dessert

Choice 2: 2 tablespoons low-sodium tomato sauce on 1 cup whole-wheat pasta with 2–3 meatballs (do not add cheese to this meal), fresh berries

Choice 3: 4–6 oz. broiled or baked red snapper fillet with lemon or lime juice and 1–2 tablespoons pesto, sugar-free Jell-O for dessert

Choice 4: Broiled salmon steak or other fish with steamed broccoli and carrots, 1 cup low-fat plain yogurt mixed with berries, and sprinkled with pumpkin seasoning

Choice 5: Caesar salad with 1 boiled egg, spinach, celery, carrots, 2 oz. low-fat cheese such as mozzarella or feta, and 4 oz. either turkey or chicken, finished with apple salad with walnuts and just a touch of balsamic vinegar

Choice 6: 4–6 oz. lean steak with steamed green beans, berries for dessert

Choice 7: Chicken breast, steamed snow peas, and sweet potatoes, sprinkled with turmeric

Choice 8: Stir-fried chicken with 1 cup mixed vegetables and fresh ginger, 1 slice low-fat cheesecake topped with fresh raspberries for dessert

Choice 9: Grilled fish with salsa, grilled asparagus, sweet potatoes

Choice 10: 8 oz. skinless roasted turkey, 1½ cups oven-roasted vegetables, with 1 glass grape juice or red wine, 1 handful mixed nuts without salt

Choice 11: 4 oz. broiled salmon or trout, 1 baked sweet potato, asparagus, ¾ cup strawberries

Choice 12: 2 cups whole-wheat pasta topped with 1 cup marinara sauce, 1 cup diced vegetables, 1 tablespoon grated low-fat Parmesan cheese

Choice 13: 3 oz. skinless roasted chicken breast, ½ cup mashed sweet potato, ½ cup green beans sprinked with sliced almonds and dried cranberries, 1 grapefruit

Choice 14: 4 oz. broiled salmon or trout, ½ cup corn, 2 cups green vegetables

Choice 15: 4 oz. broiled wild salmon stir-fried with 1 cup
   vegetables, 1 cup couscous

HEALTHY SNACKS

Have at least two snacks a day, the first between breakfast and
lunch, and the second between lunch and dinner.

Yogurt with nuts, berries, or ¼ teaspoon of organic maple syrup

Bananas with some cinnamon or cocoa powder, or just plain

1 or 2 soft-boiled eggs with some baby carrots

2 oz. low-fat cheese with grapes, green apple, and mixed raisins

5 whole-wheat sesame-seed crackers with olive oil for dipping

Yellow, orange, and green pepper strips

When Gary first walked in my door, it was immediately clear why
he'd come to see me. At six foot one and three hundred pounds, Gary
was obese. He experienced chronic hypertension, a heart murmur, attention and concentration difficulties, shortness of breath, constipation,
sweating, headaches, dizziness, depression, and anxiety. His Braverman
Nature Assessment showed that he had a strong dopamine deficiency as
well as a severe GABA deficiency.

I put Gary on the Rainbow Diet and told him that once he got his
weight under control, many of his other symptoms of brain chemical
imbalance would resolve. Gary needed to supplement his diet with rice
bran fiber and a once-a-month growth hormone shot to enhance his
metabolism. Just one month later, Gary returned with a normal blood
pressure and a loss of thirty-eight pounds. His chest pains had
decreased, and his depression had lessened considerably. At this point, I
told him to stay on the Rainbow Diet and supplement his efforts with
my GABA-enhancing agent Brain Calm. A month after that, Gary was
down to 250 pounds, his blood pressure was still normal, and he
reported that his headaches had gone away. Five months later, Gary's
weight was down to 210, and he was committed to losing even more.

By following the Rainbow Diet, you are taking an important step
on the path to total health. This diet is for the rest of your life, so that

you can eat delicious, healthy foods on a regular basis. By following this eating plan, the occasional chocolate cake, pizza, or pasta meal will not upset your entire system.

THE HELPING HANDS OF CES

Electricity powers the brain and the body, so it makes perfect sense to me to use electrical current to balance brain function. The third and final component of the Braverman Prescription is the CES device. Cranial electrical stimulation, or CES, is a therapeutic procedure that can be done in the privacy of your own home, using mild battery-powered electronic stimulation for the treatment of anxiety, depression, and insomnia. CES alters the abnormal electrical connections that can occur with drug or alcohol abuse and other organic brain diseases as well as normalizing other dysfunctional brain patterns. In short, CES helps us balance our brain waves.

For more than ten years I have seen the positive effects of CES on hypertension, headache, and pain relief. It's only a matter of time before CES is approved for other conditions. The CES device is particularly effective for men, who are prone to tense, restrictive, anxiety-prone health imbalances associated with the left brain. CES is safe, noninvasive, and nonaddictive, has no pharmaceutical side effects, and can be used daily. Positive results may be experienced immediately, though for some it takes up to three or four weeks. For lasting benefits, treatment should be continued at regular intervals.

POSITIVE EFFECTS OF CES

Enhanced cognition

Reduced anxiety

Reduced depression

Reduced insomnia

Reduced withdrawal symptoms

Improved brain waves

Enhanced neurotransmitter functions

Relapse prevention

Prevention of substance abuse in high-risk individuals

For example, to counteract exposure to microwave radiation and magnetic fields during the day, use a CES device for forty-five minutes every evening while relaxing, reading, or watching TV. Using a CES can help recharge neurons and promote conversion of choline to produce acetylcholine. In terms of GABA, the CES device can help an individual feel less overwhelmed—a great antidote to overextension and a contribution to a successful marriage between head and heart.

Obtaining a CES device requires a prescription from a physician. The FDA has approved CES use for anxiety, depression, and insomnia, and the U.S. Patent Office has issued a patent to me for its use—I have devised a specific method of applying the electrodes to forehead and wrist for optimal use.

Irene was a fifty-six-year-old woman who had suffered from migraine headaches for thirteen years. They had started out occurring about twice a month but had become more frequent during the last four years. She was treated by a neurologist with a variety of medications, including Elavil, Reglan, Corgard, Calan, Blocadren, Vistaril, Norgesic, and Anaprox, with only Blocadren giving some mild relief, but no great change. During these headaches she could not concentrate at all.

When I saw Irene, I immediately gave her the Braverman Nature Assessment and determined that she was a GABA nature. I took her off the other medications and put her on the seizure medication Depakote. She reported back to me that she received 90 percent relief. However, my goal is to always limit prescription medication as much as possible. A few months later I started Irene on the CES device and was able to reduce the Depakote in the first month. After using the CES device for about two months, she began to lower the Depakote further.

CONTINUING ALONG THE PATH

By following the Braverman Prescription, you can begin to stop the aging process and start leading a healthier, more productive life. Besides death and taxes, another certainty is that as we age, first we slow down, then we break down. The good news, as you've seen in this chapter, is that most pauses, if treated early enough, can be postponed for a long time, making vigorous health a lifelong state. By reactivating the brain, you can reactivate the hormones and organs in your aging body.

9

HEALING SPECIFIC SYMPTOMS

AND CONDITIONS

THE LIST OF conditions that are related to or caused by abnormal brain chemistry is enormous. I have treated over four hundred conditions, all related to brain chemical imbalances. The individual nature chapters in Part II list the symptoms and conditions that are commonly affected by each of the biochemicals.

In my practice, I have seen that there are certain conditions that most often occur for each of the biochemical natures. This chapter covers these illnesses and gives instructions for a variety of treatments, from a traditional medication approach to a more holistic, alternative strategy.

If you are suffering from a particular condition that is not listed in this chapter but is listed in one of the nature chapters, please refer to that chapter for possible treatment alternatives. If your symptoms are minor, then choose one of the lifestyle treatments. If your symptoms are moderate to severe, I suggest that you see your doctor about these symptoms immediately.

You can take a proactive approach to your treatment by informing your physician about the results of your Braverman Nature Assessment. The information about your biochemical nature, as well as any significant deficiencies, will be invaluable to your doctor. With this information, he or she can properly choose which medications or treatments to prescribe for both your condition and your nature.

EVEN THE SMALLEST INFECTIONS CAN DAMAGE THE BRAIN

Just as a change in brain chemistry can change your health, poor health can change brain chemistry. Left unchecked, minor changes in brain chemistry can snowball into a significantly greater problem. For example, in order to maintain optimal health, it's important to keep your body free of infections. Even the smallest infections can affect our brain in many ways. Infections can trigger an abnormal immune response, resulting in drastic illnesses, including mental disorders and some cancers. Chlamydia, a relatively minor sexually contracted infection, has been linked to multiple sclerosis, which is an acetylcholine disease. The common flu can contribute to dopamine-linked Parkinson's disease. When you are infected with the flu, your dopamine level is diminished. That is why Parkinson's drugs such as amantadine (Symmetrel) and rimantadine (Flumadine), which build dopamine, can help to alleviate the flu.

This means we must learn to take care of our brains and our bodies on both macro and micro levels. Not only is it important to follow the Braverman Prescription for total, lasting health, it's equally important to consistently practice good hygiene, especially when you are around infected individuals.

DISEASES OF DOPAMINE DEFICIENCY

A deficit in any of the four primary neurotransmitters can cause a cascade of health problems. When brain chemistry is altered, you will begin to experience the negative side of the Edge Effect. Just one chemical imbalance can cause you to lose a corner of the edge, which can damage the entire physiology.

Dopamine deficiencies are all about losing control. When your dopamine levels falter, your metabolism and muscle movements become erratic. Your emotional state is affected, since you can no longer control your deepest desires, whether they are for food, drugs, or sex. When you rebalance your dopamine, you are reversing the negative side of the Edge Effect. You will regain control of your brain and body, returning yourself to the zone of good health.

ADDICTION

Addiction is defined as a repetitive, compulsive, destructive behavior that a person cannot willfully stop. It can involve a variety of substances, including drugs, alcohol, cigarettes, caffeine, carbohydrates, fat, junk food, and even codependent relationships. Learning to break addictive patterns is the most critical dimension of preventive medicine, because addictive behavior is at the root of most of our chronic diseases. For example, alcoholism leads to liver disease, and carbohydrate addiction leads to obesity.

Abnormal brain chemistry, especially when dopamine deficiencies or excesses are involved, can lead to cravings, which are the body's automatic response for temporary healing. Unfortunately, even when these cravings are met, the brain continues to require the consumption of the craved substances just to meet its minimum requirements. By constantly supplementing the brain with these craved substances, you are creating an addiction.

The classic example of a biochemically based addiction is alcoholism. Faced with an excess or deficiency of dopamine, some people will begin to self-medicate, using alcohol to quiet their brain. Alcoholics usually attribute their drinking to mood disorders such as depression and anxiety, two common dopamine-related conditions. However, although the brain will be temporarily sated, increased alcohol consumption begins to wreck the body. First it will lead to across-the-board nutrient depletion. Later it will affect the kidneys and liver.

Conditions that create an alcohol craving, such as depression and anxiety, can be overcome with lifestyle changes, including nutritional supplements. The biochemical cause of alcohol and drug abuse may be helped by correcting deficiencies of B vitamins (especially niacin and thiamine), magnesium, zinc, and several antioxidants and amino acids (tryptophan and phenylalanine). These are all dopamine-friendly supplements.

Even minor addictions must be thwarted in order to obtain total brain and body health. For example, almost everyone I know loves to eat chocolate. This indulgence has been used for centuries to self-medicate our low moods. Because of its pseudo-elevating effect, chocolate was once called the "food of the gods." Chocolate contains phenylethylamine, which is known for causing emotional highs and lows associated with mood swings, love, pleasure, and indulgence. Chocolate also contains the chemical theobromine, which triggers the release of endorphins in the brain and works as a natural antidepressant.

However, we all know that too much chocolate is bad for you, from your waistline to your teeth. Worse, with continued intake, addicting substances can deplete endorphins and will not lead to their restoration. Addictions can be treated with natural techniques such as my dopamine Brain Energy supplement program.

OBESITY

Obesity has become one of our most critical health problems. Roughly 64 percent of all adults in the United States are either overweight or obese—meaning they are more than 20 percent above their ideal body weight. Obesity has been linked directly to such significant health problems as diabetes, cardiac problems, hypertension, sexual dysfunction, and depression.

Obesity stems from both your genetic makeup and a variety of chemical imbalances. A deficiency in any of the primary neurotransmitters can lead to obesity; however, I have found that the best treatment for this disease is a dopamine program. Dopamine agents are stimulants. They increase the power of your bodily electricity, and they also increase your metabolism, so that you turn the foods you eat into fuel more efficiently. A dopamine diet, which is a high-protein diet, gives you necessary amino acids that aid in digestion and keep you feeling full, even hours after you have eaten.

Amanda was five feet five inches tall and weighed 190 pounds when I began seeing her. Amanda was able to use dopamine biochemistry treatments, aerobic exercise, the CES device, and hormone replacement therapies to practically double her metabolic rate. This extra boost to her metabolism helped her to lose seventy pounds in just six months, and keep the weight off.

PARKINSON'S DISEASE

The classic disease of dopamine deficiency is Parkinson's disease, which affects approximately one million Americans. Parkinson's disease begins as a dopamine deficiency, which wears out the brain both biochemically and electrically. Scientists now believe that as dopamine is depleted in Parkinson's patients, the brain's neurons may be rendered dysfunctional. This causes irreversible physical damage to the brain and impairs its ability to powerfully distribute its electricity.

Parkinson's disease is a neurological disorder that causes not only characteristic changes in motion (including rigidity, tremors, slowness, and loss of reflexes that help maintain posture) but cognitive decline as well. This slowdown can be directly correlated to a decrease of brain power. In a neuroelectrical sense, the brain of a Parkinson's patient functions like that of a one-hundred-year-old, regardless of the person's biological age.

The main therapy for Parkinson's disease is the amino acid L-dopa, which converts into dopamine in the brain. Parkinson's patients also respond to a range of neurotransmitter and dopamine support agents, with an emphasis on amino acids. Methionine has been a particularly useful amino acid, as it stimulates the body's own production of L-dopa. Tyrosine and phenylalanine mimic the effects of L-dopa in the brain. Tryptophan may serve to inhibit tremors.

Numerous studies have been undertaken on other nutrients that may be helpful in treating Parkinson's. For example, antioxidants, including vitamins E and C, counter damage by free radicals and may prevent the progression of Parkinson's by slowing the damage to brain nerves. Parkinson's patients should also receive specific dietary instructions. For example, they could benefit from a vegetarian breakfast and lunch, with fruits as a main component, which would minimize the blocking of amino acid absorption and the conversion to dopamine. There are patients with Parkinson's disease who come into my office unable to walk whom we are able to restore to full health.

DISEASES OF ACETYLCHOLINE DEFICIENCY

Acetylcholine is a natural moisturizer that helps cells retain fluid and maintains the membrane coatings of cells. All acetylcholine deficiencies lead to dehydration, and once this corner of the edge is lost, you can experience a cascade of physical conditions that all relate to a literal drying out. Once your brain starts to dry out, it can no longer regulate your immune system properly. It also triggers the joints to dry out prematurely, so the brain calls on calcium resources in the bones to add moisture to the system, thereby drying up the bones as well. If you can keep your brain young, you can manage this aging process and even regain use of atrophied muscles and bones. I have seen patients who have gone from bed-bound lives to regaining full movement. By restoring your edge you can have strong bones, strong joints, and a healthy body.

ARTHRITIS

Acetylcholine controls moisture levels throughout the body. When you are experiencing an acetylcholine deficiency, moisture evaporates and dryness occurs, followed by inflammation. This three-part process is the predecessor of arthritis. Arthritis flares up when joint lubrication is lost and the body loses its ability to relubricate, or maintain, healthy joints. Interestingly, when the brain loses its moisture, cognitive deterioration begins. This is why as we age, cognitive deterioration and bone loss often occur simultaneously.

Arthritis can be treated by following an acetylcholine-boosting regimen, including hormone therapies, proper diet, supplements, and exercise. I have had great success using the supplement methionine, which has been compared to ibuprofen for the treatment of arthritis, only without the gastrointestinal side effects.

OSTEOPOROSIS

Osteoporosis is a painful and debilitating condition in which the damage can be done decades prior to the first actual bone fracture. Not only does bone density loss affect the architectural support of your body, but the injuries that can occur from this disease may erode the quality of your life, since the simplest tasks become difficult to manage once you lose bone strength. Eighty percent of all patients with osteoporosis are women, yet one third of all men also will experience its symptoms by the age of seventy-five.

Bone is living tissue composed of a soft, porous center encased in a hard outer surface. Osteoporosis occurs when the porous center becomes far less dense than the outer surface, causing the bone to literally collapse on itself. This is one reason why older people tend to lose height with age. Their vertebrae, composed almost entirely of the softer, more porous bone, shrink in size as it loses density.

There are many risk factors affecting bone health, including over-consumption of alcohol, cigarettes, caffeine, and sodium and undercon-sumption of dietary calcium. When you are experiencing early signs of this disease, any osteoporosis treatment plan should first address revers-ing these lifestyle choices. A preventive program would include additional nutritional supplementation to enhance levels of calcium and other minerals, including boron and strontium. Weight-bearing, anaerobic exercises are also recommended to promote further bone building. Brief daily exposure to the sun is also important, as it promotes the con-version of vitamin D to calcitriol, essential for building bone health.

If you are experiencing symptoms of osteoporosis, you should seek medical attention immediately. You can work with your doctor to develop a customized acetylcholine-building program that can slow bone degra-dation and offer pain relief. I usually treat osteoporosis patients with a combination of the supplements mentioned above, as well as hormone replacement therapy to correct bone deficits that have already occurred. I use a combination of growth hormones and natural estrogen, proges-terone, and testosterone to raise the activity of bone-building cells.

MULTIPLE SCLEROSIS

Multiple sclerosis is a relatively common chronic neurological disorder. Beginning as a series of benign symptoms, it can lead to an incapacitat-ing condition. It often attacks people between twenty and forty (with a higher incidence in women), frequently in the optic nerve, spinal cord, and brain. MS occurs as lesions or holes form on the myelin sheaths (formed in part from acetylcholine) found around the nerves in the brain, slowing down conduction, with potentially devastating effects on the functions of neuronal circuits in the brain and spinal cord.

Classic symptoms of MS include weakness, numbness, impaired vision, double vision, trouble swallowing, intention tremor (trembling when you intend to do something, as opposed to Parkinson's, which is associated with a rest tremor), trouble walking, impairment of deep sen-sation, bladder dysfunction, and altered emotional responses. MS can induce a tingling electrical-like feeling down the back and inner thighs, as well as unsteadiness in walking. Depression is the most common psychological symptom of MS. In addition, there are frequently impairments in memory, attention, and conceptual reasoning.

Often the most successful treatment of MS uses a multidisciplinary approach. These treatments and techniques can both arrest the disease as well as manage the symptoms. Use of strong antidepressants, such as phenelzine (Nardil) and selegiline (Eldepryl), which help enhance dopamine by blocking enzymes that break down dopamine, might slow the progress of the disease. Hormone replacement therapy, using only naturally synthesized prescriptions, may offer MS patients some relief from their condition. MS is associated with a depletion of the adrenal glands' hormone DHEA, and so by adding low concentrations of DHEA, some symptoms may be alleviated.

Dietary changes may also affect the chronic course of this disease. High intake of polyunsaturated oils (e.g., safflower oil) has frequently been demonstrated to slow the progression of MS. I encourage my MS patients to increase their intake of raw fruits and vegetables and to stay away from chemical preservatives and processed foods. They avoid tap water and limit their intake of eggs. Also, new studies have shown that vitamin D has a powerful effect on the aging brain, especially for MS patients, given that it preserves the membranes of the body, such as myelin. Vitamin D can be found in fortified milk, as well as in supplement form and through brief, regular exposure to sunlight.

My MS patients are instructed to follow our acetylcholine and GABA programs, the latter because GABA calms patients and their nervous systems, and in this way many patients have eliminated a good number of the condition's symptoms. For example, Ellen, a forty-four-year-old woman, had been suffering from MS for almost fifteen years. She walked with a cane and was having difficulties with her vision. She was taking oxybutynin (Ditropan) to treat a bladder problem and had been treated with traditional MS drugs such as baclofen (Lioresal) and steroids without success. She suffered from constipation, depression, severe fatigue, and numbness in her limbs.

I first put Ellen on a low-fat, high-complex-carbohydrate diet. I gave her evening primrose oil and fish oils (for their anti-inflammatory and anti-blood-clotting effects), an antioxidant, a multivitamin, antidepressants, and amino acids. I told Ellen that her health was in her hands. Even though a dismal prognosis often accompanies a diagnosis of MS, she did not have to believe that she would be disabled. She was invited to cultivate a hopeful outlook. Sure enough, once the antidepressants began to work, her overall outlook improved. She threw away her cane, and her numbness subsided dramatically. Her ability to move and her energy level improved, with a nearly complete remission of fatigue. To this day she continues with her antidepressants, and has more than a 60 percent remission of her overall MS symptoms.

DISEASES OF GABA DEFICIENCY

GABA deficiencies can cause a cascade of anxiety, which almost always results in some type of pain. When you are anxious, your body reacts—the blood vessels clamp down and blood pressure increases. Or your signals misfire and you get chronic pain. GABA deficiencies can cause one illness after another, until balance is restored. When you get your GABA controlled, your body returns to its natural rhythm.

CHRONIC PAIN

One in three Americans suffers from some kind of chronic or recurring pain. Seventy-six million of us experience back pain; thirty-six million endure the pain of arthritis; twenty million have migraine headaches. Pain is a symptom of a greater problem, one often caused by a brain chemical deficiency. Most likely, those who experience chronic pain have a GABA deficiency, where the brain's electrical rhythm is not sent to the body in a smooth flow.

Most doctors will prescribe sedating painkillers, antidepressants, or drugs such as oxycodone (OxyContin) to their patients with chronic pain. While these painkilling drugs are effective, they are also addictive. To date, there are four million OxyContin addicts who use this drug to mask their pain. What's more, none of these treatments resolves the problem of a GABA deficiency.

I treat chronic pain patients with a more natural approach. I usually prescribe a combination of nutrients, including 5-hydroxytryptophan; D, L-phenylalanine; methionine; and fish oils; depending on their level of GABA deficiency. This combination is particularly effective for those who suffer from arthritis and migraines. Other nutrients such as vitamin B_6, zinc, and manganese can help deal with the stress that often accompanies pain. Researchers have found that chronic pain is often both a mental and physical condition.

SEIZURES

Seizures occur on a continuum that begins with anxiety, depression, insomnia, and panic. All of these symptoms are related to a GABA deficiency, as they occur when the brain has lost its natural rhythm. Some seizures occur after a head trauma, which can produce GABA imbalances. During a seizure, you may experience symptoms ranging from involuntary outcries to urinary or bowel incontinence, a sinking feeling, increased anxiety, tongue biting, hand tremors, and epileptic convulsions. Seizures can also be limited to specific areas of the body. For example, subjective tinnitus (a spontaneous auditory condition) often entails metallic ringing, blowing, buzzing, clanging, popping, roaring, or nonrhythmic beatings in one or both ears. When this occurs, your ears are probably experiencing a localized seizure.

I have found that inositol and my GABA supplement Brain Rhythm are the cornerstone treatments for anyone who is prone to seizures. Seizures are extremely difficult to control nutritionally, although studies suggest that vitamin E may help. Other nutrients such as vitamin B_6, magnesium, and taurine may have some beneficial effects. Common nutrients, such as calcium and magnesium, may also help.

HYPERTENSION

Hypertension is the prime contributor to coronary heart disease and stroke, yet in itself it is often nothing more than irritable vascular syndrome. When hypertension occurs, your arteries begin to harden and your blood pressure rises. Fifteen to 20 percent of Americans have hypertension. Left untreated, not only can it damage your heart, but it can also cause harm to your kidneys, lungs, eyes, nervous system, and brain.

I have helped hundreds of patients lower their blood pressure to a normal level and keep it that way for years. My course of treatment does not rely solely on hypertension drugs, but rather incorporates natural techniques that will eventually replace the drugs. With all medications my goal is to get my patients to a point where they can be drug-free.

The amino acid taurine is an important part of the hypertension treatment equation. Taurine is a sulfur-containing amino acid. Adults can synthesize their own taurine: it can be found in the brain, heart, breast, gallbladder, and kidneys, where it plays important roles in the health of these organs. Taurine can also be found in high concentrations in animal and fish protein. Like GABA, taurine has a calming effect, and taurine is the second most important inhibitory neurotransmitter in the brain. This inhibitory effect explains its anticonvulsant and anti-anxiety properties. Megadoses of taurine have been proven to be useful in many patient groups, including those with anxiety or a variety of heart-related conditions, such as myocardial infarction, congestive heart failure, elevated cholesterol, supraventricular arrhythmias, and hypertension.

Along with taurine, I usually prescribe a nutrient program containing fish oils, garlic, evening primrose oil, magnesium, and vitamin B_6. My patients follow the Rainbow Diet along with the GABA regimen in order to lower their cholesterol and blood pressure.

Kevin was a fifty-five-year-old man with a history of heart conditions. He had already experienced his first heart attack and wanted to make sure that he did not have another one. At six feet two inches and 172 pounds, Kevin was underweight, and he was not in good health. When Kevin came to see me, his cholesterol was at 234. To control blood pressure he was taking diltiazem (Cardizem), which, combined with his physical condition, left him feeling sluggish all the time.

I put Kevin on the Rainbow Diet, as well as a nutrient program consisting of fish oils, evening primrose oil, niacin, and my hypertension multivitamin. In three weeks his cholesterol fell from 234 to a much more reasonable 130. What's more, his blood pressure normalized at 120/70. Six weeks later he had a cholesterol level of 114, and his blood pressure had dropped further. At this point I took him off the Cardizem, and he has never looked back. Today Kevin is fit, healthy, and medication-free. What's more, his energy and well-being have greatly improved.

DISEASES OF SEROTONIN IMBALANCES

When we lose sleep, we forfeit all of the other positive dimensions of the Edge Effect. A deficit here forces every other internal system out of whack: you lose your dopamine sense control, your acetylcholine cognitive abilities to manage life, and your overall GABA stability. Productive sleep, governed by the biochemical serotonin, gives you the freedom and abilities to balance the other corners of the edge at night, so that you can experience the Edge Effect during the day: the zone of total brain/body energy, the Zen of body and brain stability, and the nirvana awareness of higher consciousness.

SLEEP DISORDERS

Sleep is a central predictor of your overall health. Sleeping gives your brain a chance to resynchronize every night. I cannot say it more plainly: sleep and relaxation behavior predict longevity.

A serotonin imbalance produces sleep disorders, although sometimes GABA imbalances can cause disturbances as well. By building up your serotonin, not only will you sleep better, but you also allow your dopamine and acetylcholine to replenish. This increase can help get you to the Edge Effect: you will have more power and energy all day long. What's more, new research suggests that good sleep may be essential in maintaining a healthy immune system.

There are many general rules for getting good sleep, including avoiding sleeping pills, sleeping at regular times, getting regular physical exercise, limiting naps during the daytime, quitting smoking, avoiding caffeinated beverages, and limiting television, computer time, and stimulating reading material before bedtime. Yet despite adhering to these rules, many people simply cannot sleep well.

The first step in solving a sleep disturbance is making small lifestyle adjustments. You can try taking a warm bath or at least a footbath before going to bed, having a cup of soothing herb tea, and keeping your bedroom cool and well ventilated. If these don't work, nutrients can help, and unlike most drugs, they do not result in exacerbation of daytime psychiatric problems, like depression. The nutrient tryptophan at dinner and bedtime is effective in starting sleep and, in some cases, keeping a person asleep. Niacin and niacinamide prolong the tryptophan effect. Melatonin and GABA also can contribute to quality sleep. Vitamin B_6, pantothenic acid, and other B vitamins also increase dream recall and promote satisfying sleep. Inositol and vitamin C can be helpful too.

If drugs are necessary, anti-anxiety drugs, antidepressants, or anticonvulsants—such as alprazolam (Xanax), clonazepam (Klonopin), gabapentin (Neurontin), trazodone (Desyrel), or sinequan (Doxepin)—and/or antihistamines are best. Occasionally, major tranquilizers such as thioridazine (Mellaril) are necessary. However, the problem with using prescription drugs as sleep aids is that they are addictive. Instead, I recommend using the CES device, which I find to be the best treatment of insomnia developed to date.

SUGAR CRAVINGS AND TYPE 2 DIABETES

Sugar cravings in those suffering from hypoglycemia and depression have multiple origins. One biochemical study suggests that decreases in serotonin cause us to crave sugar. Serotonin is made from tryptophan, and tryptophan supplementation frequently decreases sugar craving. High-protein diets, featuring a high tryptophan to carbohydrate ratio, also reduce sugar cravings.

Sugar cravings can lead to type 2 diabetes, a metabolic disorder that causes a chronically elevated blood sugar level. Unlike type 1 diabetes, which is an insulin-dependent condition occurring most commonly in children, type 2 diabetes is linked to increased intake of sugar and simple carbohydrates and obesity. Previously, type 2 diabetes was classified as an adult disease, but with the surge in childhood obesity, doctors are diagnosing patients at every age group with this condition.

Through its effect on your blood sugar levels, diabetes has the potential to trigger other seemingly unrelated yet significant medical conditions, including foot ulcers, kidney failure, depressed immune function, eye diseases, permanent nerve damage, circulatory problems, hypertension, and heart disease.

Glucose tolerance factor (GTF) has been reported to help regulate blood sugar. This compound is beneficial for both diabetics and hypoglycemics. GTF contains chromium, which is frequently reduced in the plasma of patients with sugar cravings. Inositol may also quell carbohydrate cravings. All diabetics must follow a strict diet that eliminates foods with high sugar content. This diet should be discussed with your own physician.

Type 2 diabetics become insulin resistant, and as they age they lose their growth hormone (with advancing years all of our hormone production slows down). Efforts to improve insulin production naturally include herbal supplements such as *Gymnema sylvestra,* or nutrient supplements such as zinc and the B complex vitamins. I have seen complete reversals of type 2 diabetes with many of my patients, even those with severe forms of this disease. For example, I once treated a woman who came to me with dopamine deficiency and life-threatening type 2 diabetes, and within six months of beginning a strict dopamine diet and nutrient program, she had completely normal sugar levels. Often when patients are low in dopamine they feel tired, so they use carbohydrates and sweets as energy quick fixes; soon this food becomes part of their daily diet, leading to weight gain and possibly diabetes due to high amounts of sugar in the blood and inadequate amounts of insulin. Many times I recommend a dopamine diet for breakfast and lunch and a GABA diet at dinner to calm down diabetic patients.

ANOREXIA, BULIMIA, AND SEXUAL ADDICTION

Anorexia, bulimia, and sexual addiction are all related to serotonin imbalances. Although eating and sex may at first seem very different, these two pleasure-inducing acts are intricately related, and problems with their control can be caused by serotonin deficiencies. When examined more closely, both of these problems are related to synchrony: anorexia and bulimia occur when the signals of the brain to eat are out of sync, and sexual addiction occurs when signals for sexual appetite are miscommunicated.

All three of these syndromes are classified as psychological disorders, and if you are experiencing any amount of binge eating, purposely regurgitating your food, or feeling an constant, overwhelming desire for sexual relations, you should seek psychological help immediately. A physician can prescribe selective serotonin reuptake inhibitors (SSRIs) such as paroxetine (Paxil) and fluoxetine (Prozac) to control these syndromes. Besides therapy, I often recommend natural serotonin-boosting agents, including my Brain Mood formula, to help resynchronize the brain.

MULTINATURE ILLNESSES

Many illnesses can occur from a combination of nature deficiencies. Other illnesses can be caused by any one of several deficiencies. For example, obesity is usually a disease stemming from a dopamine imbalance, but it can also be a result of cravings produced through acetylcholine, GABA, or serotonin deficiencies. The following short list highlights many of the most common multinature illnesses and effective treatment alternatives.

PMS

Most women experience minor symptoms related to their menstrual cycle, such as bloating, headaches, backaches, cramping, and general irritability, all of which signal a minor biochemical deficiency. However, with premenstrual syndrome, or PMS, symptoms including depression, mood swings, feelings of aggression or violence, migraine headaches, and joint and muscle pain, among others, indicate that the levels of both GABA and serotonin are unbalanced.

Serotonin-enhancing medications such as fluoxetine (Prozac) and GABA-enhancing medications such as Xanax can be helpful. However, try to avoid medications and the dependency they create. I have successfully treated hundreds of women with natural agents, such as GABA-friendly inositol and serotonin-friendly tryptophan. You can try any of the natural or lifestyle programs described for these two natures. I have also found that the CES device is very helpful for PMS. Interestingly, the 3M Corporation markets a CES-like device that is meant solely to treat PMS.

STROKE

About fifteen million ministrokes and half a million full-blown strokes occur every year. Nearly 150,000 people die of strokes annually, and an additional 300,000 people are left crippled to some extent.

Strokes are caused either by blocked blood vessels in the brain (ischemic stroke) or by ruptures in the brain's blood vessels (hemorrhagic stroke). Most are caused by the former. Symptoms include sudden weakness or numbness to the face, arm, or leg (usually one side of the body), loss of speech or trouble talking or understanding speech, dimness or loss of vision (particularly in one eye), unexplained dizziness, unsteadiness, frequent falls, or sudden severe headache.

A physical exam is of minimal value in finding who is going to have a stroke. High cholesterol is somewhat predictive. An MRI tells you if someone is already having a stroke. The best stroke predictor is regular duplex carotid artery scanning and ankle brachial index, tests that carry up to an 86 percent accuracy rate. In order to avoid stroke, common

recommendations include lowering blood pressure, lowering cholesterol, and following a well-balanced, low-fat diet. If you have diabetes,
keep it under control. Don't smoke or drink alcohol. GABA treatments
to reduce anger and frustration can also prove effective, as all sorts of
stress, ranging from retirement issues to marital problems, have been
associated with higher rates of stroke, even in nonhypertensive patients.

The nutrient most associated with reducing the extent of the damage done by a stroke is carnitine, probably because of its relationship with
acetylcholine. Carnitine works by building up acetylcholine, the main
memory compound, in the stroke-damaged brain. This enables the brain
to shift memories from damaged cells to cells in undamaged parts of the
brain, to store new information, and to create new memories. This action
is analogous to shifting information on a computer: the brain is simply
transferring information to another disk or to a different hard drive.

The toxic effect of stroke occurs as a result of the release of calcium
into the cells, as well as an excessive release of the amino acids glutamate
and aspartate, which are neurotoxic in moderate to large quantities.
GABA-friendly nutrients can help protect cells against these factors.
Studies have documented the benefit of vitamin A in reducing stroke
damage, as well as possibly the general category of antioxidants, which
include vitamin E, selenium, cysteine, vitamin C, and beta-carotene.
There may be some additional benefit in giving low dosages of Dilantin
or other antiseizure medications to patients after a stroke, because following a stroke as many as 5 to 15 percent of patients may experience a
seizure. In France, studies have shown that *Ginkgo biloba* has also been
thought to be helpful in cerebral insufficiency. Primary and secondary
prevention of stroke includes the use of ginger, onion, garlic, cayenne
pepper, fish oils, aspirin, and willow bark. These natural supplements
are especially beneficial to patients who have already had a stroke
caused by blocked brain blood vessels.

SEXUAL DISORDERS

The four natures all play an important role in sexual function. Dopamine
controls libido, aggression, and power. When people lose interest in sex,
they are usually experiencing a dopamine deficiency. When a patient is
sad or blue and has no sex drive, antidepressants such as Wellbutrin and
Effexor are great for increasing sexual interest. An equally effective over-

the-counter treatment that combats psychogenic impotence is the herb yohimbine, which is also a dopamine-related compound. Any of the other dopamine-enhancing nutrients can be used as a sexual enhancer, including my Brain Energy formula.

A loss of acetylcholine affects your creative consciousness. In terms of sexual issues, less-creative feelings inhibit your ability to view yourself as a sexual person. Furthermore, as acetylcholine controls the moisture levels in the brain and body, a loss of this biochemical will affect women sexually because as they age they lose their ability to lubricate the vagina. Acetylcholine does not impact sexual performance as powerfully as dopamine; rather, its impact is felt over the course of a lifetime. For example, young people have the highest amount of sexual activity because their acetylcholine is at its peak, while older people usually experience a drop-off in sexual activity. Use acetylcholine-enhancing compounds to produce a general increase in sex drive.

When it comes to addressing sexual problems, doctors tend to look at GABA remedies to treat sexual anxieties or to enable people to relax in order to enjoy sexual relations. For example, an alcoholic drink or two will immediately relax you and help you overcome performance anxiety. We do it all the time in our culture when we engage in normal sexual mating rituals. We go out, we have a drink, and all of a sudden we get in touch with our suppressed sexual energy. GABA-friendly medications such as Xanax act in the same way. Nutrients such as inositol can also help calm the mind and body so that you can enjoy sexual relations.

In the case of premature ejaculation, doctors have been able to help men prolong erections by tapping into the serenity factor of serotonin. Essentially, all cases of premature ejaculation respond to serotonin-enhancing drugs. As we know, SSRI antidepressants such as Paxil, Celexa, Prozac, and Zoloft build serotonin. In addition, patients experiencing sexual problems frequently respond to tricyclic antidepressants that raise serotonin levels, such as Anafranil.

Women and men who have an excess of serotonin often have trouble having orgasms. If they have too much dopamine, on the other hand, they are quicker to have an orgasm, which can be a problem for men.

Alex was a sixty-year-old man who came to me complaining of anxiety, tension, and lack of sexual activity. Alex looked to be overweight, and a routine physical examination revealed mild hypertension and mild enlargement of the prostate. A Doppler ultrasound test, which detects blockages of the arteries and veins, indicated a significant loss of blood flow to the brain. His Braverman Nature Assessment revealed a severe dopamine deficiency. Blood testing revealed low testosterone.

I treated Alex with Androderm (a testosterone patch), Paxil (to address his anxiety, verbal memory loss, and overall brain function decline), DHEA, and nitroglycerine cream—which acts as a vasodilator. One month into his treatment, the patient reported improved sexual function, specifically stating that his erections had returned and were quite satisfactory. Additionally, he'd lost ten pounds and simply felt better.

The sexual Edge Effect occurs when all four of your primary neurotransmitters are balanced or enhanced. When your dopamine is high, you experience strong sex drive. When your acetylcholine is high, you are sexually aware and creative. Your body becomes better lubricated: it is easier for you to have an orgasm, and a woman might be able to have multiple orgasms. When your GABA is high, your mind is connected to your sexuality. Sex comes easily: there is no tension, frigidity, or premature ejaculation. When your serotonin is high, you have an ideal duration of intercourse, neither too short nor too long. You have a fluid connection between your sexual fantasies and your real life. When the balanced brain hits these four peaks, you will reach new states of sexual experience.

THE BALANCED-BRAIN ADVANTAGE

As you can see, so many medical conditions are the result of a brain that's out of balance. The story of all illness is imbalance at the edge. Over the past twenty-five years, I have seen almost every major medical condition in my patients and have reversed them all by balancing the brain. The proper selection of nutrients and hormones to enhance all four neurotransmitters triggers a cascade that completely reverses or puts into remission all types of illnesses. Simply put, the Edge Effect makes a powerful difference.

You can return to total health. By following the suggestions with regard to your primary nature you can regain your edge. And by enhancing all of the natures, you can prevent further aging, reverse your current conditions, and experience the full Edge Effect.

10

IMPROVING YOUR MEMORY

As we age, many of us fear losing our memory. The threat of Alzheimer's is particularly scary: in 1997 alone, 2.3 million people as young as age sixty were diagnosed with this disease. Most people worry about forgetting names, telephone numbers, and where they put things.

The good news is that most memory complaints are not problems with memory at all but can be attributed to a biochemical loss that also shows up as anxiety, depression, illness, or emotional disturbances. For example, the tip-of-the-tongue syndrome, in which you forget things but feel as though you're on the verge of recalling them, is really just a symptom of anxiety. What's more, Alzheimer's, anxiety, and memory loss are not inevitable consequences of aging. Rather, they are concrete indications of brain chemical deficiencies, and they can all be reversed.

When mild deficits are uncovered early, nature-specific remedies can be used to postpone the ravages of senility. If you experience any problems with memory, don't ignore them. As we age, we lose many of the brain's nerve connections, but we do not lose brain cells. Some studies even suggest that we can grow new brain cells and reconnect disconnected brain cells.

PERCEPTION AND MEMORY

There are two universal truths regarding our ability to remember: memory is not always accurate, and memories do not last forever.

Memory is affected by perception, feeling, and experience. As we age, we remember events differently. Memories of traumatic childhood events are frequently distorted because of their emotional content, and false memories can easily occur—the reality of a memory is extremely difficult to establish without independent confirmation. If you ask individuals to remember events from childhood at age fifty-five and then at age seventy, their answers vary greatly.

The full effect of perception depends considerably on how an event is experienced and filtered through memories, emotions, and fantasies, because perception is colored by past experiences, associated memories, and concurrent social inputs. For example, how a person remembers a trip to New York City depends in part on the person's feelings, experiences, and beliefs about the city. People visiting New York for the first time and know of it primarily as a city of tall buildings may remember the skyscrapers; others who previously lived there and disliked it may retain a perceptual memory of a dirty, crowded city of scowling faces.

The intensity of perceptions depends on an individual's sensitivities, mood, level of anxiety, substance use, and health. If you ask ten of your friends to watch an event together and report on the details, all ten will have slightly different takes because they all perceive things uniquely. For example, clinically depressed people often describe colors as faded, conveying a sense that the world looks washed-out, even though their capacity to recognize and distinguish specific colors is unchanged.

THE FOUR TYPES OF MEMORY

Every one of us is born with a range of perceptual and memory abilities. There are four distinct types of memory that can reflect a particular biochemical imbalance: working memory, immediate memory, verbal memory, and visual memory.

Working memory involves the ability to concentrate quickly or take in information or stimuli that are verbally or visually presented. When a stimulus is presented to the brain, your working memory either quickly records it or doesn't. Working memory involves bringing together old and current data. If you are overloaded with the latter, the brain will dump older memories to make room for new ones. Long-term memory correlates with working memory: if you can absorb information initially, you will also be able to store it. The functions of working memory include motor control, concentration, problem-solving skills, planning, retention of knowledge, and initial registration, all of which are regulated by the frontal lobes and the neurotransmitter dopamine.

Immediate memory is a short-term effect—lasting only about thirty seconds—that occurs when a stimulus is presented but before it has been recorded in long-term memory. It is difficult to distinguish where working memory ends and immediate memory begins. Immediate memory comprises both verbal and visual memories. It is helpful for mastering simple daily activities and is an indication of one's learning capabilities and basic alertness. Immediate memories are briefly stored in the parietal lobes, which are regulated by acetylcholine.

Verbal memory is necessary for storing sounds, words, and stories. For example, listening to a lecture and later recalling exactly what was said demonstrates good verbal memory. The temporal lobes, which are regulated by GABA, store memories of written or verbally presented information.

Visual memory involves the ability to absorb and retain information such as faces, colors, shapes, designs, symbols, and your surroundings. People who can drive to a location after having been there only once demonstrate excellent visual memory. The serotonin-producing occipital lobes control visual and sensory training and connect with the immediate memory of the parietal lobes.

A memory begins with the reception of information controlled by the parietal lobes and the neurotransmitter acetylcholine. If brain speed is optimum, the memory will be passed on and processed in the frontal lobes, which are powered by dopamine. Memory decline starts at the beginning: if we cannot receive information, we cannot process or store it. Signs of memory loss are therefore characterized by slowed brain speed and abnormal power and metabolism. Identifying what your particular memory problem stems from is as easy as identifying your nature. Not surprisingly, the two are closely linked.

THE BRAVERMAN
MEMORY TEST

Many of the elements of the Braverman Memory Test are comparable to the Wechsler Memory Scale (WMS), and the Randt Memory Test, recognized standards for testing short-term memory and attention. There are six parts to this test. Please set time aside to complete the entire test in one sitting. You can take as much time as you like to complete the tests. For many of the sections it will be beneficial to have someone else assist you. Make sure that you are well rested before you take this memory test. Follow all directions carefully and record your answers in this book. If you believe that you are already experiencing the early stages of memory loss you might want to photocopy the test pages so that yhou can take the test again at a later date, after you have been following my healing program.

After completing all of the tests you will be able to see if your answers were correct. You will tally your points at the end of the tests to determine your score. Ideally, set aside one hour or complete each part before resting.

PART 1: STORIES
(Auditory and Immediate Memory)

Instructions: Carefully read each of the following stories one time. This test would be more effective if you could have someone else read the stories to you slowly. After each story, write down the answers to the questions. Do not read the questions before you read the story, and do not refer back to any part of the story in order to answer the questions. If you can't answer any question immediately, skip the question entirely: do not revisit the questions missed once the test is finished. When you have answered all the questions, proceed to the next story.

STORY 1

Jacob Welch is an eight-year-old Cub Scout whose goal is to earn the recruiter badge from his Cub Scout pack. He has been working to recruit other classmates at his school, Walker Elementary. One of Jacob's classmates, Andy Parkinson, came to the sign-up night at St. Paul's Church with his father. At the next Cub Scout pack meeting on Monday, October 19, Jacob received the recruiter badge. His parents were so proud of him that they took him out after the meeting for his favorite dessert, two scoops of chocolate ice cream in a sugar cone.

Questions for Story 1

1. What is the Cub Scout's name? _____

2. How old is he? _____

3. What is his goal? _____

4. What school does he attend? _____

5. What is his friend's full name? _____

6. Who accompanied Andy to the meeting? _____

7. What was Andy doing at the meeting? _____

8. What month was the next Cub Scout meeting? _____

9. What date was the next Cub Scout meeting? _____

10. What happened at the next meeting? _____

11. Who was at the meeting with Jacob? _____

12. What was the reaction of Jacob's parents? _____

13. What did they take him to get after the meeting? _____

14. How many scoops does Jacob like? _____

15. What was the flavor? _____

16. Was it in a cup? _____

17. If not, what was it in? _____

STORY 2

A young girl was walking to school on a Monday as she passed a brick building that was under construction. Five men were there tearing the building down and were working on the seventh floor. As she turned onto Lexington Street, the girl heard what sounded like kittens crying. She went up to the building and saw three kittens huddled in a corner. The kittens were white and black, and there was no mother cat in sight. The girl could not leave the kittens at the construction site, so she put them in her backpack and took them to school. At the end of the day, she sold the kittens to classmates for $10 each.

Questions for Story 2

1. Was the story about a boy or a girl? _____

2. What day of the week was it? _____

3. Where was she walking to? _____

4. What did she pass on her way to school? _____

5. What was the building made of?_____

6. What was happening to the building? _____

7. How many men were working on it? _____

8. What street did she turn onto? _____

9. What did she hear as she turned the corner? _____

10. What did she find at the construction site? _____

11. How many were there? _____

12. What color were they?_____

13. Was the mother there? _____

14. Where did she take them?_____

15. How did she take them? _____

16. What did she do with them?_____

17. How much did she sell them for? _____

STORY 3

Missy and Daniel McKinnon have owned the Healthy Coffee Shop on the corner of Wilson Street and Benson Street for the past twenty years in rented space. In November the building was sold to another person by the name of Bart Styles. Bart decided to increase the rent by more than $200 per month. Missy and Daniel decided the rent was too expensive and found a new location on River Street. Their shop will be open for business on January 14, and they will be having specials on coffee and special health shakes made of strawberries.

Questions for Story 3

1. What are the first and last names of the shopkeepers? _____

2. What is the name of their store? _____

3. Where was the store located? _____

4. How long had the store been at that location? _____

5. Did they own the building where the store was? _____

6. When was the building sold? _____

7. What was the name of the man who bought it? _____

8. What did the new landlord do? _____

9. What did Missy and Daniel do in reaction to the rent increase?

_____

10. Where will the new store be located? _____

11. What month will they be open for business again? _____

12. What date will they open for business again? _____

13. Will they be serving all their food at the regular price? _____

14. Will they be having specials on salads? _____

15. What are they having specials on? _____

16. Do they serve health shakes? _____

17. What are the shakes made of? _____

STORY 3—SECOND RECALL

Return to page 207 and reread Story 3, then answer the next set of questions. Do not read the questions before you read the story, and do not reread any part of the story to answer the questions. The test will be more accurate if someone else can read the story aloud to you.

Questions for Story 3—Second Recall

1. What are the first and last names of the shopkeepers? _____

2. What is the name of their store?   _____

3. Where was the store located? _____

4. How long had the store been at that location? _____

5. Did they own the building where the store was? _____

6. When was the building sold? _____

7. What was the name of the man who bought it?   _____

8. What did the new landlord do? _____

9. What did Missy and Daniel do in reaction to the rent increase? __

_____

10. Where will the new store be located? _____

11. What month will they be open for business again? _____

12. What date will they open for business again?   _____

13. Will they be serving all their food at the regular price? _____

14. Will they be having specials on salads? _____

15. What are they having specials on? _____

16. Do they serve health shakes? _____

17. What are the shakes made of?   _____

PART 2: OBJECTS
(Visual and Immediate Memory)

On the following pages you will see three sets of 24 objects each; set 1 contains the reference objects. You are going to look at each object in the first set for two seconds. To do this most effectively, take a sheet of paper and cut a one-inch square out of the middle. Then place the opening over one picture at a time, until you have viewed all of the objects. The goal is to become familiar with each object within the two seconds and then move on to the next one. Then you may begin to view the second set of objects. This time, look at the entire two-page spread at once. The goal of the test is to identify the objects you saw previously. Use the grid below to record your answers after you have viewed the second set of objects. As you view each object, answer yes if you remember seeing it previously and no if you do not. Repeat the test on the third set of objects. Use the answer sheet below to record your answers.

Answer Sheet
Circle Y or N to indicate your answer.

Set 2

a) Y / N	g) Y / N	m) Y / N	s) Y / N
b) Y / N	h) Y / N	n) Y / N	t) Y / N
c) Y / N	i) Y / N	o) Y / N	u) Y / N
d) Y / N	j) Y / N	p) Y / N	v) Y / N
e) Y / N	k) Y / N	q) Y / N	w) Y / N
f) Y / N	l) Y / N	r) Y / N	x) Y / N

Set 3

a) Y / N	g) Y / N	m) Y / N	s) Y / N
b) Y / N	h) Y / N	n) Y / N	t) Y / N
c) Y / N	i) Y / N	o) Y / N	u) Y / N
d) Y / N	j) Y / N	p) Y / N	v) Y / N
e) Y / N	k) Y / N	q) Y / N	w) Y / N
f) Y / N	l) Y / N	r) Y / N	x) Y / N

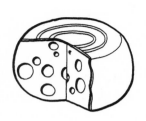
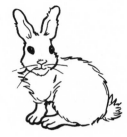

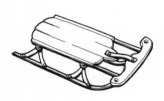
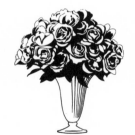
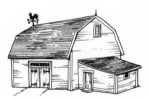

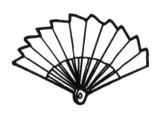
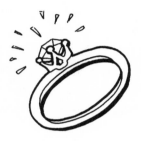
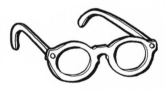

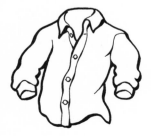
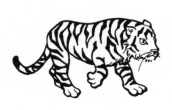
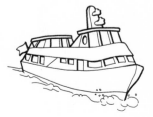

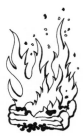
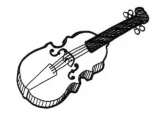
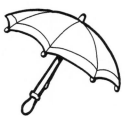
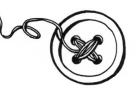
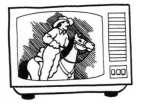
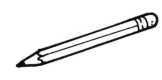
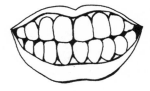
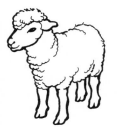
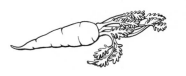
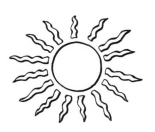
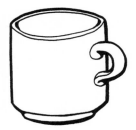
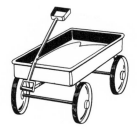

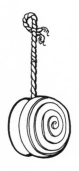

a)

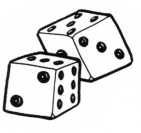

b)

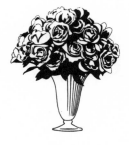

c)

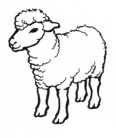

g)

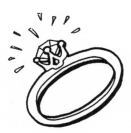

h)

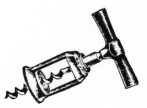

i)

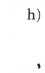

m)

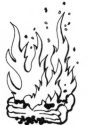

n)

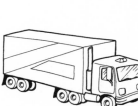

o)

s)

t)

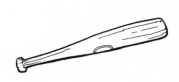

u)

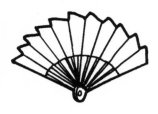

d)

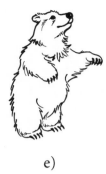

e)

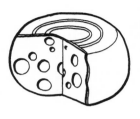

f)

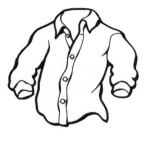

j)

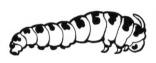

k)

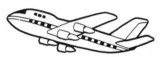

l)

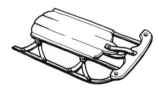

p)

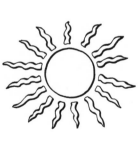

q)

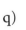

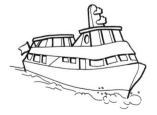 r)

v)

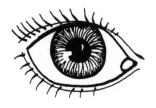

w)

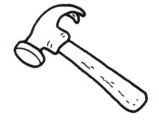

x)

a)

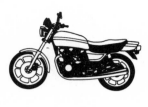

b)

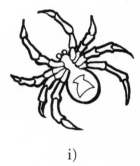

c)

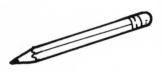

g)

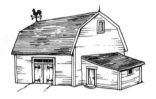

h)

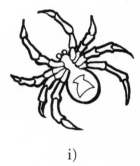

i)

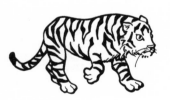

m)

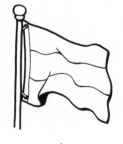

n)

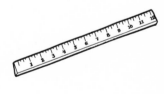

o)

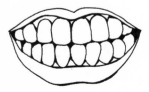

s)

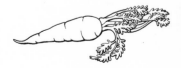

t)

u)

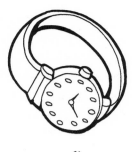

d)

e)

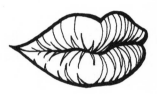

f)

j)

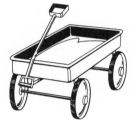

k)

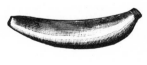

l)

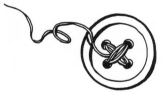

p)

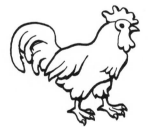

q)

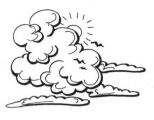

r)

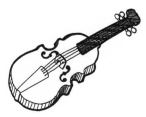

v)

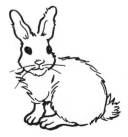

w)

x)

PART 3: PAIRS
(Auditory and Immediate Memory)

Instructions: This test is most effective if you have someone assist you. You are going to try to remember what words are matched together. Have your assistant read the eight word pairs in the trial column carefully and slowly, at a rate of approximately one pair every three seconds. Then have your assistant turn to the recall column and read the first word of each pair. It is your job to recall the second word of each pair.

For example, *dog-apple* is a word pair. In the recall column you will see **dog** _____. If you have an assistant, say *apple* aloud, and your assistant will write it down. If no assistant is available, read these words to yourself aloud, and then cover the pairs in the trial column with a sheet of paper and fill in the blanks at right as best as you can.

This test consists of four trials to recall the eight pairs in different orders. Once you have finished the first trial, move on to the next.

Trial 1

car-stripe

wasp-tree

snake-rainbow

garage-magazine

circle-stairs

rabbit-popcorn

daisy-box

giraffe-mirror

Recall 1

1. garage _____

2. snake _____

3. circle _____

4. daisy _____

5. giraffe _____

6. car _____

7. wasp _____

8. rabbit _____

Trial 2

circle-stairs

giraffe-mirror

wasp-tree

car-stripe

snake-rainbow

garage-magazine

rabbit-popcorn

daisy-box

Recall 2

1. giraffe _____

2. wasp _____

3. snake _____

4. daisy _____

5. circle _____

6. rabbit _____

7. garage _____

8. car _____

Trial 3

daisy-box

rabbit-popcorn

circle-stairs

snake-rainbow

giraffe-mirror

wasp-tree

garage-magazine

car-stripe

Recall 3

1. wasp _____

2. circle _____

3. car _____

4. daisy _____

5. giraffe _____

6. snake _____

7. garage _____

8. rabbit _____

Trial 4	Recall 4
rabbit-popcorn	1. circle _____
car-stripe	2. daisy _____
circle-stairs	3. wasp _____
wasp-tree	4. rabbit _____
daisy-box	5. giraffe _____
snake-rainbow	6. garage _____
garage-magazine	7. snake _____
giraffe-mirror	8. car _____

PART 4: PICTURES
(Visual and Immediate Memory)

Instructions: Look at each picture for ten seconds. Study all of the minute details. Try to remember as much as you can about the picture. Then turn the page and answer the questions pertaining to that scene. Give yourself about five seconds to answer each question. If you don't know the answer after five seconds, move on to the next question.

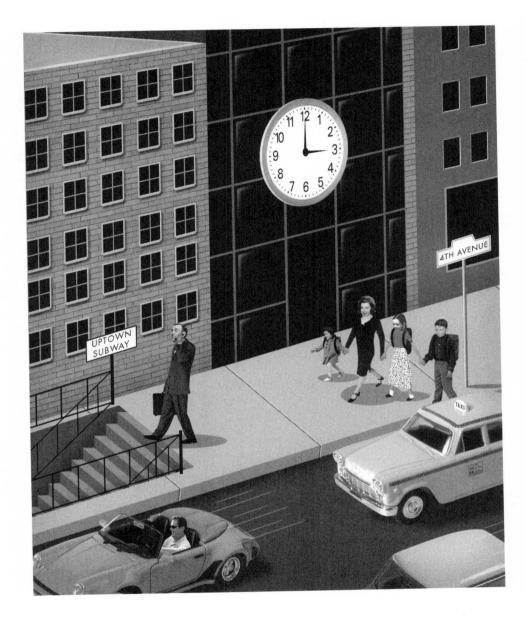

Picture A

Questions for Picture A

1. How would you describe the scene? _____

2. How many people are walking down the street? _____

3. What time is it? _____

4. How many children are in the scene? _____

5. What are they carrying? _____

6. Is the woman's hair dark or light? _____

7. What is the man holding? _____

8. What is the name of the street? _____

9. How many buildings are in the scene? _____

10. What type of train is the man going to take? _____

11. How is the man dressed? _____

12. How many taxicabs are in the picture? _____

13. How many signs are on the sidewalk? _____

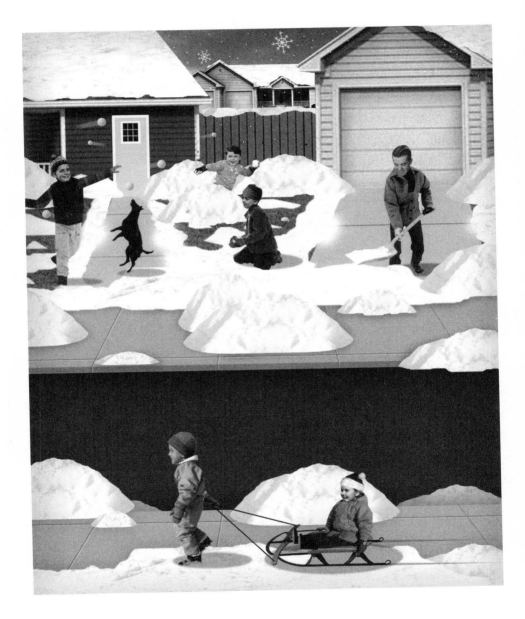

Picture B

Questions for Picture B

1. Where does the scene take place? _____

2. What is going on in the picture? _____

3. How many children are in the picture? _____

4. What is the little girl doing? _____

5. How many children are wearing hats? _____

6. What are the boys doing? _____

7. What is the dog doing? _____

8. What is the man doing? _____

9. Is it snowing? _____

10. Does the girl seem happy? _____

11. What kind of hat is the girl wearing? _____

12. How many houses are in the picture? _____

13. Do any of the houses have fences around them? _____

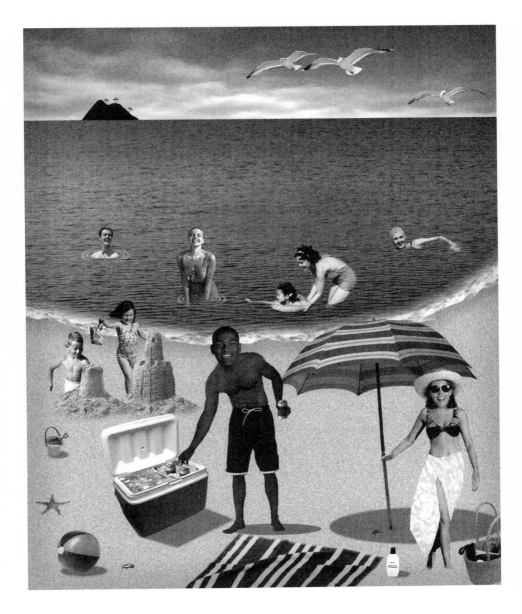

Picture C

Questions for Picture C

1. How would you describe the scene?_____

2. What is the woman on the beach doing? _____

3. Are there clouds in the sky? _____

4. What else is in the sky? _____

5. What is the man doing? _____

6. What are the children doing? _____

7. Does the man's bathing suit have stripes?_____

8. Whose sandcastle is bigger? _____

9. What is the woman on the beach wearing? _____

10. How many towels are laid out? _____

11. What is the man holding? _____

12. Is there a dog in the picture? _____

13. How many people are in the water?_____

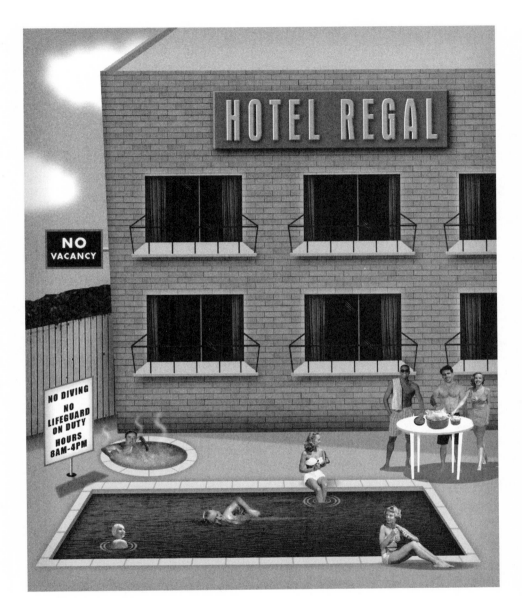

Picture D

Questions for Picture D

1. What is the name of the hotel?_____

2. How many stories is the hotel?_____

3. What activities does the hotel have? _____

4. Are there any vacancies at the hotel?_____

5. How many balconies overlook the pool?_____

6. What are the pool rules? _____

7. What time does the pool close? _____

8. How many people are in the middle of the pool? _____

9. What is the man in the pool doing? _____

10. Is there a lifeguard on duty? _____

11. What are the people at the table doing? _____

12. Are they drinking? _____

13. How many clouds are in the sky? _____

PART 5: NUMBERS
(Working Memory)

Section A: This test will be more effective if you have someone else read it to you slowly. However, if that is not possible, please read the directions for taking this test alone.

Instructions if you are taking this test with an assistant: Have the assistant read each sequence one at a time. Repeat back the sequence in the exact order you heard it. The assistant should record your answer in the space provided. If you miss two consecutive sequences, move on to the next exercise. Calculate your total number of correct sequences.

Instructions if you are taking this test alone: Read each number sequence once, then cover it with a piece of paper and write down the sequence from memory in the space provided. Continue to work down the list until you miss two consecutive sequences. Calculate your total number of correct sequences and move on to the next exercise.

1. 8-3   ___-___

    2-9   ___-___

2. 6-9-2   ___-___-___

    6-1-7   ___-___-___

3. 5-7-3-4   ___-___-___-___

    8-6-0-9   ___-___-___-___

4. 1-8-6-3-9   ___-___-___-___-___

    2-7-4-5-6   ___-___-___-___-___

5. 7-2-5-9-4-8   ___-___-___-___-___-___

    0-8-3-1-2-5   ___-___-___-___-___-___

6. 2-9-8-3-5-7-6   ___-___-___-___-___-___-___

    3-9-8-6-5-2-7   ___-___-___-___-___-___-___

7. 8-7-9-0-2-6-1-4   ___-___-___-___-___-___-___-___

    8-2-7-3-9-5-4-0   ___-___-___-___-___-___-___-___

8. 3-5-2-7-9-6-2-3-0   ___-___-___-___-___-___-___-___-___

    7-2-8-4-1-3-0-2-6   ___-___-___-___-___-___-___-___-___

Section B: Read the sequence of numbers, following the same instructions as in Section A. However, write down or repeat the numbers *in the reverse order.* For example, sequence 1-2 would be written down 2-1. If you miss two consecutive sequences, please move on to the next exercise.

1.   1-3   ___-___

      2-9   ___-___

2.   2-8-7   ___-___-___

      5-0-8   ___-___-___

3.   9-7-8-6   ___-___-___-___

      7-4-2-4   ___-___-___-___

4.   1-8-6-3-9   ___-___-___-___-___

      9-1-2-6-8   ___-___-___-___-___

5.   7-2-5-9-4-8   ___-___-___-___-___-___

      0-8-3-1-2-5   ___-___-___-___-___-___

6.   3-0-4-2-7-1-8   ___-___-___-___-___-___

      3-5-4-1-2-8-0   ___-___-___-___-___-___

7.   6-9-7-4-1-3-7-8   ___-___-___-___-___-___-___

      8-2-7-3-9-5-4-0   ___-___-___-___-___-___-___

PART 6: NUMBERS AND LETTERS
(Working Memory and Concentraton)

Instructions: You are going to arrange the letters and numbers that you read or hear (if you have an assistant) in a certain order. The first sequence contains one letter and one number. The trick is that when you recall the sequence you must always *put the number first.* For example, both H-5 and 5-H would be recorded as 5-H.

The sequences will become increasingly difficult, involving more than one number and letter. Continue arranging the numbers before the letters. Both the numbers and the letters should be in ascending order. For example, 2-G-4 should be recorded as 2-4-G; 8-Z-D-2 should be recorded as 2-8-D-Z. If you miss two sequences, stop.

1.   R-1   ___-___

2.   D-2   ___-___

3.   7-T   ___-___

4.   G-P-2   ___-___-___

5.   K-9-3   ___-___-___

6.   A-5-P   ___-___-___

7.   R-9-2-1   ___-___-___-___

8.   C-3-4-Z   ___-___-___-___

9.   7-N-2-U   ___-___-___-___

10.   2-E-6-B-4   ___-___-___-___-___

11.   X-1-C-8-H   ___-___-___-___-___

12.   7-Y-2-6-A   ___-___-___-___-___

13.   M-7-E-4-Y-2   ___-___-___-___-___-___

14.   Q-9-I-8-K-3   ___-___-___-___-___-___

15.   4-R-6-B-2-S   ___-___-___-___-___-___

16.   R-3-J-1-U-5-E   ___-___-___-___-___-___-___

17.   Y-7-D-3-N-4   ___-___-___-___-___-___

18.   W-9-P-2-S-6   ___-___-___-___-___-___

19.   G-1-E-7-N-2-P-6   ___-___-___-___-___-___-___-___

20.   D-1-J-4-K-2-L-7   ___-___-___-___-___-___-___-___

BONUS SECTION
(Passive Memory Recall)

After you finish the six parts to the test, see if you can recall the names of each section. Write them down in the spaces provided.

Part 1 _____

Part 2 _____

Part 3 _____

Part 4 _____

Part 5 _____

Part 6 _____

ANSWER KEY

Part 1: Give yourself 1 point for each correct answer. Record the number of correct items in the space below.

Story 1

1. Jacob Welch
2. Eight years old
3. To earn the recruiter badge
4. Walker Elementary School
5. Andy Parkinson
6. Andy Parkinson's father
7. Sign-up night
8. October
9. The nineteenth
10. Jacob was awarded the recruiter badge
11. His parents
12. They were proud of him
13. To get ice cream
14. Two
15. Chocolate
16. No
17. Sugar cone

Story 1 total (1–17): _____

Story 2

1. A girl
2. Monday
3. To school
4. A building
5. Brick
6. It was under construction/being torn down
7. Five men
8. Lexington Street
9. Crying kittens
10. Kittens
11. Three
12. Black and white (½ point for only one color)
13. No
14. To school
15. She put them in her backpack
16. She sold them to her classmates
17. $10 each

Story 2 total (1–17): _____

Story 3

1. Missy and Daniel McKinnon
2. The Healthy Coffee Shop
3. On the corner of Wilson Street and Benson Street
4. Twenty years
5. No
6. November
7. Bart Styles
8. He increased the rent by over $200 per month
9. Found a new location
10. River Street
11. January
12. The fourteenth
13. No

14. No
15. Coffee and health shakes (½ point for only one right)
16. Yes
17. Strawberries

Story 3 (first recall) total (1–17): _____

Story 3 (second recall) total (1–17): _____

Total for Part 1 (0–68): _____

Record the total score on the raw score sheet on page 236.

Part 2: Give yourself two points for each correct answer.

Set 2

a. N___	g. Y___	m. Y___	s. Y___
b. N___	h. Y___	n. Y___	t. N___
c. Y___	i. N___	o. N___	u. N___
d. Y___	j. Y___	p. Y___	v. Y___
e. N___	k. N___	q. Y___	w. N___
f. Y___	l. N___	r. N___	x. N___

Set 3

a. Y___	g. Y___	m. Y___	s. Y___
b. N___	h. Y___	n. N___	t. N___
c. N___	i. N___	o. N___	u. Y___
d. N___	j. Y___	p. Y___	v. Y___
e. N___	k. Y___	q. N___	w. N___
f. Y___	l. N___	r. N___	x. Y___

Total score for Part 2 (0–48): _____

Record the total score on the raw score sheet on page 236.

Part 3: Give yourself 1 point for each correct answer.

Recall 1	Recall 2	Recall 3	Recall 4
1. magazine	1. mirror	1. tree	1. stairs
2. rainbow	2. tree	2. stairs	2. box
3. stairs	3. rainbow	3. stripe	3. tree
4. box	4. box	4. box	4. popcorn
5. mirror	5. stairs	5. mirror	5. mirror
6. stripe	6. popcorn	6. rainbow	6. magazine
7. tree	7. magazine	7. magazine	7. rainbow
8. popcorn	8. stripe	8. popcorn	8. stripe
Total (0–8):___	**Total (0–8):___**	**Total (0–8):___**	**Total (0–8):___**

Total score for Part 3 (0–32): _____
Record the total score on the raw score sheet on page 236.

Part 4: Give yourself 1 point for each correct answer.

Picture A	Picture B
1. City street/sidewalk/afternoon	1. On a residential street
2. Five	2. People shoveling/playing
3. Three o'clock	3. Five
4. Three	4. Being pulled on a sled
5. Backpacks	5. Four
6. Dark	6. Having a snowball fight
7. A cell phone/briefcase	7. Jumping
8. 4th Avenue	8. Shoveling
9. Three	9. Yes
10. Subway	10. Yes
11. In a business suit	11. Knit
12. One	12. Three
13. Two	13. Yes
Picture A total (0–13): _____	**Picture B total (0–13):** _____

Picture C

1. The beach/seashore
2. Setting up an umbrella
3. Yes
4. Seagulls
5. Taking something out of cooler
6. Swimming/building sandcastles
7. No
8. The girl's
9. A bikini top and a wrap
10. One
11. A can
12. No
13. Five

Picture C total (0–13): _____

Picture D

1. Hotel Regal
2. Two
3. Swimming/hot tub
4. No
5. Six
6. No diving
7. 4 PM
8. Two
9. Swimming laps
10. No
11. Snacking
12. No
13. Two

Picture D total (0–13): _____

Total score for all Part 4 pictures (0–52): _____

Record the total score on the raw score sheet on page 236.

Part 5: Give yourself 1 point for each correct answer.

Section A

1. 8-3
    2-9
2. 6-9-2
    6-1-7
3. 5-7-3-4
    8-6-0-9
4. 1-8-6-3-9
    2-7-4-5-6

5. 7-2-5-9-4-8
    0-8-3-1-2-5
6. 2-9-8-3-5-7-6
    3-9-8-6-5-2-7
7. 8-7-9-0-2-6-1-4
    8-2-7-3-9-5-4-0
8. 3-5-2-7-9-6-2-3-0
    7-2-8-4-1-3-0-2-6

Section A total 0–16): _____

Section B

1. 3-1

    9-2

2. 7-8-2

    8-0-5

3. 6-8-7-9

    4-2-4-7

4. 9-3-6-8-1

    8-6-2-1-9

5. 8-4-9-5-2-7

    5-2-1-3-8-0

6. 8-1-7-2-4-0-3

    0-8-2-1-4-5-3

7. 8-7-3-1-4-7-9-6

    0-4-5-9-3-7-2-8

Section B total (0–14): _____

Total score for Part 5 (0–30): _____

Record the total score on the raw score sheet on page 236.

Part 6: Give yourself 1 point for each correct sequence.

1. 1-R

2. 2-D

3. 7-T

4. 2-G-P

5. 3-9-K

6. 5-A-P

7. 1-2-9-R

8. 3-4-C-Z

9. 2-7-N-U

10. 2-4-6-B-E

11. 1-8-C-H-X

12. 2-6-7-A-Y

13. 2-4-7-E-M-Y

14. 3-8-9-I-K-Q

15. 2-4-6-B-R-S

16. 1-3-5-E-J-R-U

17. 3-4-7-D-N-Y

18. 2-6-9-P-S-W

19. 1-2-6-7-E-G-N-P

20. 1-2-4-7-D-J-K-L

Total score for Part 6 (0–20): _____

Record the total score on the raw score sheet on page 236.

Bonus Section: Give yourself 1 bonus point for each correct test title.

Part 1: Stories

Part 2: Objects

Part3: Pairs

Part 4: Pictures

Part 5: Numbers

Part 6: Numbers and letters

RAW SCORE SHEET FOR
BRAVERMAN MEMORY TEST

Individual Raw Scores

Part 1: Stories (0–68): _____ (Auditory/Immediate Memory)

Part 2: Objects (0–48): _____ (Visual/Immediate Memory)

Part 3: Pairs (0–32): _____ (Auditory/Immediate Memory)

Part 4: Pictures (0–52): _____ (Visual/Immediate Memory)

Part 5: Numbers (0–30): _____ (Working Memory)

Part 6: Numbers and letters (0–20): _____ (Working Memory/
Concentration)

Bonus Section: titles (0–6): _____ (Passive Memory Recall)

1. Add the raw scores for Parts 5 and 6, *multiply by 2*, and write the total next to Working Memory under Grand Totals.

2. Add the raw scores for Parts 1 through 4, *divide by 2*, and write the total next to Immediate Memory under Grand Totals.

3. Add the raw scores for Parts 1 and 3, and place the total number next to Auditory/Immediate Memory under Grand Totals.

4. Add the raw scores for Parts 2 and 4 and write the total number next to Visual/Immediate Memory under Grand Totals.

5. Finally, add any bonus points you received in the Bonus Section.

GRAND TOTALS:

1. Working Memory (Dopamine) (0–100):___

2. Immediate Memory (Acetylcholine) (0–100): _____

3. Auditory/Immediate Memory (GABA) (0–100): _____

4. Visual/Immediate Memory (Serotonin) (0–100): _____

5. Bonus points (0–6): _____

Interpretation of Scores

90–100+: Genius memory capabilities—your memory is functioning at a level few can attain
75–90: Above-average memory capabilities—the minimum baseline of normal memory functioning
60–75: Average memory capabilities—can indicate the possibility of an early deficiency, because most of us experience a deficiency in at least one of biochemicals at all times
35–60: Below-average memory capabilities—a sign of an existing memory deficiency that needs to be addressed
0–35: Poor memory capabilities—a sign of an existing memory deficiency that needs to be addressed

If your score was lower than you would like, do not be discouraged. There could be many reasons why your memory is not currently functioning well. Just remember that memory deficiency can be helped and, most important, it can be reversed.

WHEN DOES MEMORY FAIL?

The majority of all memory lapses are for names: those of our friends and acquaintances, famous people, and those not truly germane to our everyday life. Generally speaking, forgetting names is not much of a problem and is a normal part of our brain's mental functioning, due to the fact that we have only a limited storage area for memory. True memory problems present themselves as difficulties in speaking, reading, and writing, and as dramatic changes in personality. These are not quaint consequences of getting older—they are all early signals of cognitive decline.

As you age, the production of your biochemicals and their related hormones diminishes, potentially affecting your ability to remember. However, you should not be experiencing a failure to remember what should be familiar places and events more than once every few months until you reach the age of sixty. Forty percent of people have declining memory, or memory dysfunction, beginning at age fifty, yet some of us experience a decline in overall memory ability as early as age twenty. Many of us experience our first "senior moments" by the age of forty or forty-five, when our brain begins to lose its processing speed.

THE MANY CAUSES OF MEMORY LOSS

There are multiple physiological changes in the brain that are associated with the loss of memory and mental deterioration. No matter what age you are, a decline in memory is a signal that you are experiencing the negative side of the Edge Effect. When memory loss occurs, your brain chemicals are imbalanced. Acetylcholine is the biochemical most directly involved with memory loss.

Acetylcholine promotes two important functions: brain speed and brain moisture. Changes in brain speed mark the process of memory loss. When our brain speed slows, we cannot think as quickly, and we lose the ability to recall events, directions, or names stored in our working memory. Our immediate memory is also affected, as we lose the ability to process information from immediate to working memory. As little as ten to twenty milliseconds of lost processing speed spells the difference between optimal and suboptimal brain functioning. Remember, memory is processed as a wave and a particle; as the wave slows down, the individual particles are dropped.

The causes of a loss of brain speed are a lack of moisture and the subsequent damage to the brain's information highway. Neurons begin to lose some of their chemical firepower, and neuronal connections are short-circuited by a buildup of plaque (clumps of damaged neuronal material mixed with a sticky protein called beta amyloid), the breakdown of the insulating layer that covers neurons, and the loss of cerebrospinal fluid. These underlying physical changes cause cognitive decline.

Many acetylcholine-related medical conditions also can contribute to memory loss. Significant memory loss can occur rapidly with multiple sclerosis and in seizure patients, both of whom are suffering from the same loss of myelin sheathing. Patients with attention deficit disorder have memory processing problems due to this bumpy acetylcholine highway. Infections and inflammation, including encephalitis and HIV, affect attention and reaction time. An HIV patient may have good recognition memory but poor recall memory.

Brain speed is also directly affected by declines in the other three neurotransmitters. A dopamine deficiency and its related energy loss in the brain can manifest itself as a weakened working memory. The extra stress put on the brain to make up for the loss of power also consumes additional acetylcholine. Drug abuse, addiction, and neuropsychiatric disorders such as schizophrenia are also linked to dopamine-related memory loss.

GABA deficiencies are often signaled by chronic pain. Severe pain causes memory loss, as inadequate support from painkillers lowers GABA levels, which monitor overall brain rhythm. When brain rhythm goes, additional acetylcholine is used up. Mentally, GABA-related irregular brain rhythms indicate a memory interference that can be due to either anxiety or depression. Physically, GABA plays a role in epilepsy, which can cause memory loss and amnesia.

Serotonin deficiencies cause the brain to receive inadequate rest. Temporary memory losses occur with constant use of over-the-counter medications such as antihistamines, flu medicines, and antidiarrhea treatments, which can damage memory by affecting the sleep cycle. Over the long term, abnormal brain symmetry can lead to serious sleep disorders, which in turn cause memory interference. Lack of sleep also contributes to depression and/or trauma, which can also impair memory.

MEMORY LOSS AND THE PAUSES

As we age, our bodies produce fewer hormones, which leads to brain pauses. We produce less growth hormone between ages thirty and fifty, less estrogen and testosterone by ages forty or fifty, less DHEA between thirty and sixty, and possibly less progesterone by age sixty. These pauses can all cause memory loss. For example, a deficiency in melatonin leads to interruptions in the sleep cycle, leaving memory storage damaged; low progesterone leads to increased brain anxiety, which is destructive to memory; growth hormone deficiency stunts brain cell growth.

HOSPITAL PROCEDURES

Hospital procedures, such as bypass surgery or even something as common as general anesthesia, can also damage memory. Researchers tell us that invasive procedures for saving the heart frequently mean losing memory. For example, studies have shown that five years after bypass surgery, 42 percent of patients suffer from cognitive decline. Virtually any surgery is a memory challenge and can start the cycle of memory loss.

ALZHEIMER'S DISEASE: THE ULTIMATE
NEGATIVE EDGE EFFECT

Alzheimer's disease is one of the most frightening prospects of old age. *Alzheimer's* is a term used to describe a collection of dementias and dementia symptoms beginning with cognitive or memory deterioration and often definitively diagnosable only by autopsy, which reveals the disease's characteristic plaques, neuronal tangles, and shrinkage of the brain. Alzheimer's disease is often referred to as brain failure, the disintegration of brain function. Alzheimer's has many stages, which begin in the temporal lobes with subtle, short-term verbal and later visual memory changes. In the most positive cases, it never progresses beyond memory loss. In the worst ones, it leads to the complete breakdown of all physical systems, including digestive and metabolic functioning, vision, and speech.

All Alzheimer's patients experience deterioration of their myelin sheaths, which causes plaques, or clumps of damaged neuronal material, along the acetylcholine highway in the brain. This is the same problem that occurs with multiple sclerosis, except that with Alzheimer's the myelin sheaths are lost in the brain only, rather than in other parts of the peripheral nervous system. The most common causes of dementia are hypertension, cigarette use, heart attack, diabetes, and high cholesterol. Cerebrovascular disease can cause ministrokes, which in turn cause considerable cognitive decline. Some individuals will have neurofibrillary tangles in the brain, or abnormally twisted protein fibers, a particular sign of Alzheimer's. Cognitive failure can be exacerbated by smoking. The most common reversible causes of change in mental state and Alzheimer's and other dementias are depression, a deficiency in vitamin B_{12}, and Parkinson's disease.

Alzheimer's is the total loss of the Edge Effect. Both multiple sclerosis and Alzheimer's are typical conditions occurring from acetylcholine deficiencies. However, a loss in any of the other biochemicals will exacerbate the loss of acetylcholine, thereby contributing to this devastating disease. As I described earlier, a dopamine deficiency speeds up your acetylcholine highway and will eventually destroy it. Lack of GABA will lead to a lack of total brain stability, which will burn out the brain faster. A serotonin deficiency might cause a lack of sleep, which will also affect the acetylcholine highway. Therefore, all diseases of the brain and body, including the aging process, ultimately contribute to the development of dementia.

WHEN MEMORY LOSS IS NOT ALZHEIMER'S

While true Alzheimer's disease occurs at an alarming rate, most patients who think they are getting Alzheimer's disease are mistaken. The onset of Alzheimer's is slow and frequently goes unnoticed. Ironically, it is anxious GABA-deficient people who will often suffer from changes in memory first, not Alzheimer's patients.

Paul was a forty-year-old man who came to see me with complaints that he was starting to experience the symptoms of Alzheimer's disease. Paul was stressed out, drinking too much coffee, working too many hours, smoking cigarettes, and generally trying to accomplish too much. He found himself unable to remember names or places and continually misplaced his keys.

Paul had a family history of Alzheimer's disease, and he tested positive for the early signs of andropause, or male menopause. His Braverman Nature Assessment showed that he did not have an acetylcholine deficiency but was very low in GABA. When we gave him the Braverman Memory Test, he tested positive for attention deficit, yet his working memory was intact. His main problems proved to be his anxiety and nervousness—the fear of getting Alzheimer's, rather than actually having it.

Paul's anxiety functioned as a siren announcing that something was wrong with his biochemical balance. He did not have classic symptoms of Alzheimer's, but his brain was slowing down. Paul's anxiety was due to a GABA deficiency, exacerbated by his working extra hard at trying to hold himself together with lower hormone levels and slower brain function than were normal for him.

I didn't treat Paul for memory loss, because that wasn't his problem. Instead, I improved his hormonal profile. I explained the benefits of GABA- and serotonin-friendly nutrients and dietary changes. I treated his andropause, because testosterone loss is closely linked to Alzheimer's. By catching Paul's problem at an early stage I was able to reverse his symptoms, including memory loss. After just one week of treatment, his anxiety abated and his memory was restored.

TREATING ALZHEIMER'S
AND BOOSTING YOUR MEMORY
WITH THE FOUR NATURES

Alzheimer's disease does not have to be life's worst-case scenario. In many ways, the way we treat Alzheimer's is similar to the way we now treat heart disease. If you can catch cardiac problems in their early stages and reverse the damage, then you can prevent heart attacks and premature death. Similarly, if you are in touch with your nature, you can recognize the early signs of memory loss before they lead to serious cognitive deterioration. I have seen many patients experience a complete reversal of memory loss when it is diagnosed and treated early.

The same treatments that I use to restore or enhance the various natures also reverse memory loss: medication, hormones, diet and nutritional supplements, exercise, lifestyle, environment, and electrical stimulation. Each of these treatment protocols is integrally linked to the four natures, because without treating brain chemical imbalances, there is no hope for anyone to improve their memory significantly. Dopamine stimulates working memory; acetylcholine helps to access memory and is responsible for speed and immediate memory function; GABA helps organize memory, particularly verbal memory; and serotonin helps with visual memory and perception.

TREATING MEMORY DISORDERS
WITH MEDICATIONS

The most serious cases of memory loss require the most powerful remedies: drugs such as donepezil (Aricept), rivastigmine (Exelon), memantine (Namenda), and tacrine (Cognex). However, these drugs are used only after the disease has progressed significantly; only then will they have any impact, at which time they can slow down the worsening of symptoms.

There is no reason to wait until you do poorly on the Braverman Memory Test or even the much simpler Mini Mental State Exam (MMSE) most physicians will use. If you catch minor imbalances early, treatment can be tailored to your nature. For example, there are other medications that seem to improve memory indirectly by working on enhancing the primary biochemicals. Diethylpropion (Tenuate) increases dopamine to give you mental energy; Klonopin increases GABA to ease anxiety, which helps you retain more information; and Zoloft is a serotonin medication that can help you to get a restful night's sleep in order to enhance cognitive recharging of the brain.

It is important to remember that drug therapy contributes only part of the edge. In order to experience a full recovery, you have to sharpen all along the edge by increasing your biochemicals through a multifaceted approach that includes nutrient supplements, hormones, and lifestyle changes. As always, medications should only be taken for the symptoms or conditions that they were initially prescribed for, and their use should always be monitored by a physician.

TREATING MEMORY DISORDERS WITH HORMONES

Hormones associated with the memory function include human growth hormone, vasopressin, DHEA, and pregnenolone, as well as estrogen and testosterone. Hormone assessment and balancing should be included in a treatment plan for severe memory impairment.

Women can experience different types of memory problems than men due to the influence of estrogen, progesterone, and other hormones. Estrogen receptors are present in several regions of the brain involved in memory and attention, including the temporal and frontal lobes. These receptors activate processes beneficial to our ability to think. Estrogen deficits leading to cognitive issues can be differentiated from other conditions through careful review of your medication history and an exam. If in fact you are experiencing memory loss due to a lack of estrogen, a personalized hormonal regimen can be constructed for you. Just as with prescription medications, it is important to be under the watchful care of a physician while taking hormones.

TREATING MEMORY DISORDERS WITH DIET AND NUTRITIONAL SUPPLEMENTS

No one needs to hear another reason to quit smoking, reduce alcohol consumption, and stay away from illegal drugs. However, put simply, if you want to preserve your mental faculties, you will do all three. Studies show that all of these habits contribute to cognitive decline. Even if advances in cloning, organ replacement, gene therapies, and nanotechnology extend the life of your body, you won't be able to enjoy the party if your brain is not functioning properly.

The biochemicals responsible for brain activity come from the foods we eat and the supplements we take. As we have discussed, memory function starts in the parietal lobes, where the neurotransmitter acetylcholine controls brain speed. Naturally enhancing acetylcholine levels when you feel that your memory is starting to fade is your first priority.

Natural supplements that are the precursors to the neurotransmitters can improve memory. Acetylcholine is synthesized by the body from choline, a B vitamin–like substance that comes from the fats in the foods we eat. However, because the digestive system is inefficient and our diet isn't always perfect, it is a good idea to supplement choline for preserving memory function. Natural formulations containing choline, in any of its many forms, along with other ingredients that support its circulation to and absorption by the brain, are a vital part of a healthy diet. Blood-flow enhancers such as quercetin and D, L-phenylalanine and herbs such as huperzine-A, *Rhodiola rosea*, and ginkgo have improved memory and focus in Alzheimer's patients. Supplements such as Cognitex, ProCog, and my Brain Youth and Brain Memory formulas are also vital to memory and cognitive functions.

The following lists of nutrients are nature-specific, and you'll see below which of the memory functions they can restore or enhance:

DOPAMINE-BOOSTING NUTRIENTS THAT IMPROVE WORKING MEMORY

- Tyrosine (used by the brain to produce dopamine and norepinephrine, has been shown to increase concentration and decrease symptoms of anxiety and depression; best used in conjunction with vitamin B_6)
- Phenylalanine (used in the manufacturing of dopamine and norepinephrine; improves learning and memory)
- L-dopa (a precursor to dopamine)
- Thiamine (a B vitamin that has a dopamine-augmenting effect)
- Chromium (a trace element that has a dopamine-augmenting effect)
- Yohimbine (an herb that has dopamine and acetylcholine effects on the brain)

ACETYLCHOLINE-BOOSTING NUTRIENTS THAT IMPROVE IMMEDIATE MEMORY AND FOCUSING

- Choline (a precursor to acetylcholine)
- Manganese (helps synthesize acetyl-carnitine)
- Acetyl-carnitine (raises acetylcholine levels in the brain)
- Phosphatidylserine (a natural preservative of acetylcholine)
- Huperzine-A (preserves choline)
- Lipoic acid (prevents breakdown of all membranes)

GABA-BOOSTING NUTRIENTS THAT IMPROVE VERBAL MEMORY AND ANXIETY-BASED ATTENTION FAILURE

- Inositol (a B vitamin that helps build GABA levels)
- Taurine (assists with GABA production)
- GABA Pentin (a modified amino acid that helps build GABA; also sold in drug form as gabapentin)
- B vitamins
- Kava
- Branched-chain amino acids (block dopamine and switch energy into physical action)

SEROTONIN-BOOSTING NUTRIENTS THAT IMPROVE VISUAL MEMORY AND REACTION TIME

- Tryptophan
- Vitamin B_6
- Melatonin
- St. John's wort
- Fish oils

OTHER NUTRIENTS TO CONSIDER

- D, L-methionine (part of the lipotropic group of amino acids; helps remove heavy metals, which are thought to cause cognitive decline, from the body)
- Pyridoxine (vitamin B_6; helps increase serotonin levels)
- Zinc (helps build the immune system; found to be deficient in children with mental retardation)
- DMAE (opens neural pathways in the brain; once it crosses the blood-brain barrier, it converts to choline)

- Pycnogenol (the brand name for pine bark extract; a powerful antioxidant that strengthens capillaries in the brain and consumes free radicals)
- Niacin (opens blood vessels and improves blood flow to brain)
- Garlic (like niacin, opens blood vessels and improves blood flow to brain)

EXERCISES TO IMPROVE MEMORY

If you don't utilize your brain's cognitive capacities, they will weaken and you will lose them. While it is true that thinking and memory will dull somewhat with age, it has recently been discovered that the adult brain can generate new cells well into old age. This means that we are capable of improving our attention and memory at any point in our lives. Across the country, performance scores on memory and attention tests are lower than they should be. Most of us don't reach our full potential due to brain-chemical imbalances and poor physical health. While some of these limitations are genetic in origin, there is plenty of room for improvement through exercise.

The more we use our mental faculties, the stronger they will be, much like a weight lifter uses curls to build up her biceps. Similarly, you can do exercises to build up your brain. None of the recommendations that follow will reverse a severe case of cognitive decline, but they are the first line of defense against memory loss, and it's never too early to apply them. It's important to note, however, that you cannot do a single bicep curl and expect to build big muscles, and the same is true of brain exercises. Only by repeating these exercises will you make progress strengthening your memory. Ideally, you should exercise the brain as much as fifty hours a month, which translates roughly to twelve hours a week, or less than two hours a day.

First, physical exercise plays an important role in mental acuity. Not only does it promote general health, which minimizes contributing factors to memory loss, but maintaining a healthy cardiovascular system ensures proper blood flow to the brain, supplying it with the raw ingredients it needs to function properly.

Most people want to improve one of the four types of memory described earlier. Study your Braverman Memory Test in detail. The low scores tell you what you need to work on. Then select exercises that are designed specifically for those areas.

To improve working memory, try your hand at memorizing names, addresses, and telephone numbers in local phone books, doing a few pages at a time. You can build your attention skills by asking a friend to recite strings of numbers and letters to you, with you repeating them back in the exact order. Crossword puzzles, brain teasers, and trivia games all flex your mental muscles.

The Braverman Memory Test itself can be used as a memory exercise. If you performed poorly on the story exercises, have someone read you a passage from another story and try to recite back the details. This will help improve your working memory as well as your verbal memory. Another exercise that might help improve your visual as well as verbal memory consists of reading the newspaper and then writing down the answers to the who, what, when, where, why, and how questions. You can pick your own stories and test yourself. Just remember to use material you have not read before. Try to recall as much as you possibly can. Drawing a design from memory is another way to check and strengthen visual memory.

TREATING MEMORY DISORDERS WITH MUSIC

Music relaxes the brain so that you can listen better. Using music to relax increases your GABA and synchronizes the left and right hemispheres. Researchers tested the benefits of music on dementia patients by employing different background noise scenarios—quiet, cafeteria noise, music—while asking them questions that would force them to concentrate deeply. The scientists found that the music playing in the background while these questions were asked significantly improved the patients' recall ability. Singing or playing an instrument yourself is an active way in which you can increase GABA.

TREATING MEMORY DISORDERS WITH CES

For general memory improvement, the CES device becomes an important tool, because it boosts all of the neurotransmitters. I've mentioned earlier in this chapter that memory loss is closely linked to anxiety, so it makes sense that when patients use CES to reduce anxiety, memory and cognition will also improve.

ATTENTION

Attention is a cognitive state associated with working memory. It is defined as withdrawing from some tasks in order to deal effectively with others. Long-term memory is extremely dependent on attention, and attention failure is frequently a sign of Alzheimer's disease and the collapse of memory.

The human brain has limited resources: if we pay attention in one area, attention to other areas may decrease. And without attention, memory storage is impossible. Attention plays a role in organizing material that can influence its later recall.

Improving attention depends upon the electrical status of the four natures, adjusting those natures, and eliminating emotional interference. In order to maximize our attention, we must maximize our nature. While memory is all about acetylcholine, attention is all about dopamine. When dopamine burns out, a person is unable to stay focused. You can improve attention skills with various dopamine-boosting supplements and techniques, including cortisol, your own version of my dopamine Brain Energy formula, and playing computerized games to improve brain speed.

Pam, a thirty-two-year-old overweight editor, came to PATH complaining that she was always exhausted, couldn't concentrate, and had severe attention problems. She also admitted that she was addicted to prescription medications that she'd begun taking for a painful chronic sports injury. She was deeply dedicated to her work, and the state of her health was affecting her ability to function in the office.

I put Pam on a program that balanced her dopamine nature, including a regimen consisting of dietary, hormonal, behavioral, and pharmaceutical elements. Pam also began using the CES device every night for one hour. Three months later, she was totally off all pain medications and had lost weight. Not only has she noticed a dramatic increase in general energy and concentration, but Pam is back to working at top speed in the office.

MEETING YOUR OWN MEMORY NEEDS

There are numerous studies of memory prodigies, such as the famous Russian mnemonists (memory artists), idiot savants, and others able to demonstrate perfect, photographic memory. Some people with a penchant for mathematics can perform lightning calculations, others demonstrate incredible auditory memory for music and speeches, and still others have the ability to memorize and recite reams of poetry.

While these remarkable powers are intriguing, there is not much call for this type of memory in our daily living. These skills do not necessarily enhance attention, intelligence, or the overall health of any human being. It is more important to have a well-rounded memory that suits each of our individualized needs. For example, a therapist requires great immediate memory. Working memory and concentration would be considered a strength for a writer or a doctor. Visual memory is useful for a movie director, and strong immediate memory suits an individual who is involved in sales. In this new electronic age, we will all be required to increase our brain speed in order to process the masses of information available to us. Those who reach and maintain the Edge Effect will be the ones to thrive in this increasingly demanding society.

11

BENDING YOUR PERSONALITY: EXPERIENCING THE FULL EDGE EFFECT

WHEN IT COMES to your personality, feeling great within your nature is common and comfortable, but you aren't experiencing the full Edge Effect. Even if you are peaking within your own nature, sooner or later you will find yourself vulnerable to certain crises or health problems. For example, if you are highly extroverted, you may find yourself in a dopamine zone, yet you will have diminished your ability to remain calm. If you let extroversion go too far, you will lose sleep, the brain will not be able to resynchronize, and a host of mental and physical illnesses can result. In order to sleep better, an extrovert might want to suppress his intensity by using the nature programs for GABA and serotonin.

As you've learned, only when the brain hits all four peaks of bio-chemical control will you reach the full Edge Effect and be able to truly rule your physical health. To reach this state, you have to balance your deficiencies and enhance your nature using the suggestions in the nature chapters. Look at your lowest scores from the Braverman Nature Assessment: those are your deficiencies, or weakest points. Those directly opposite your nature are the ones you need to build up first. For example, high dopamine and acetylcholine natures need to find balance by enhancing their GABA and serotonin. The opposite is true as well: high GABA and serotonin natures will find balance by enhancing their dopamine and acetylcholine. Then you can take control over the remaining minor natures and develop them as well.

The full Edge Effect puts you in a position to choose when to use each of the biochemicals in order to bend your brain to where you need to be at any specific point in life. Another example involves controlling your acetylcholine intuitiveness. Too much consciousness is not always a good thing. Sometimes you need to emphasize common sense, enhance the ability to form relationships, and live within the confines of reality. In these cases, this nature would need to suppress acetylcholine in order to build up the other biochemicals to emphasize extroversion and more practicality. By following the lessons outlined in this chapter, you will be able to control your personality through biochemistry.

MODIFYING NEGATIVE ASPECTS OF YOUR NATURE

The way you see yourself and the way others see you may vary widely, yet there may be more than a grain of truth in both viewpoints. Here are some ways in which your nature may be perceived by others versus how you may perceive yourself. When you compare the two, you may see why others have difficulties with you, and appreciate what you need to modify to gain a more balanced personality.

DOPAMINE NATURE

HOW PEOPLE VIEW THEMSELVES	HOW OTHERS MAY VIEW THEM
Able to rely on valid intuition	Acts on crazy hunches
Able to understand and explain complex theories	Comes up with useless ideas
Calm, not overly emotional	Aloof, distant, lacking warmth, unfeeling
Correct a high percentage of the time	Critical, faultfinding
Efficient	Doesn't care about people
Firm-minded, able to reprimand or fire if necessary	Arrogant
Objective	Heavily defended, unable to open up
Original, unique	Weird, eccentric, poor dresser

DOPAMINE NATURE (cont'd)

HOW PEOPLE VIEW THEMSELVES	HOW OTHERS MAY VIEW THEM
Powerful	Ruthless
Rational	Too abstract
Task- or goal-oriented	Unappreciative, stingy with praise for a job well done
Under control	Unrealistic

ACETYLCHOLINE NATURE

HOW PEOPLE VIEW THEMSELVES	HOW OTHERS MAY VIEW THEM
Affirming	A pushover
Caring, compassionate	Bleeding heart
Creative	Flaky, unrealistic
Empathetic	Groveling, fawning, obsequious
Expressive, expansive	Hopelessly naive
Idealistic	Illogical
Keeper of relationships, often the caretaker	Not businesslike
People person	Overemotional
Romantic	Slick, too smooth, manipulative
Social interaction expert	Smothering
Spiritual	Stuck in the past
Trusting	Too nice, Goody Two-shoes
Unselfish	Too talkative

GABA NATURE

HOW PEOPLE VIEW THEMSELVES	HOW OTHERS MAY VIEW THEM
Decisive	Always trying to set the agenda
Dependable	Blind to new opportunities
Executive type	Bossy, controlling
Goal-oriented	Drudge
Good at a sorting, weeding out, and discarding	Dull
Hard worker	Frustratingly difficult to work with
Not wasting time with impossible schemes	Judgmental

Orderly, neat	Nitpicking
Practical	Sees only the obvious
Precise	Predictable
Punctual	Uncreative
Realistic	Uptight

SEROTONIN NATURE

HOW PEOPLE VIEW THEMSELVES	HOW OTHERS MAY VIEW THEM
Able to do more than one thing at a time	Indecisive
Can deal with chaos	Unable to stick to the task at hand
Curious, welcoming new information	Resisting closure or decision
Electric	Scattered, cluttered, unfocused
Flexible, adaptable to changing circumstances	Uncontrollable, unpredictable, creating chaos
Superior ability to weigh options	Wishy-washy

TAKING ON QUALITIES
OF DIFFERENT NATURES

There are always aspects of our temperaments that we are proud of. Often these high points are overshadowed by ways in which we find ourselves lacking. However, we can apply behavioral strategies to bring out the best in each of our less dominant natures. In this way we can learn to compensate for our personality weaknesses.

Beginning on the next page are lists of exercises or ideas to make each temperament more well rounded. I call these competencies, in the sense that we are trying to achieve these personality goals. By making these behavioral changes, you will naturally increase your minor nature levels. For example, if you are a dreamy serotonin nature, by following the suggestions listed here, you can actually raise your other biochemical levels so that you will have a more balanced personality. In effect, you will be bending your personality by changing your biochemistry.

REACHING EXTROVERT COMPETENCE

For an introvert to become more extroverted, you need to add a little variety to your life. When you are learning extroverted competence, you are learning how to turn on your dopamine. Dopamine is all about power: by enhancing your dopamine, you can become a more powerful personality.

- Get involved in a group or organization such as your children's PTA, take part in a church event, or volunteer your time to a nonprofit organization or city agency. By becoming active with others, you will increase your dopamine and your acetylcholine levels and train your brain to exert more dopamine and acetylcholine behaviors.

- Add a little variety to your life by working on a few things at one time, not giving too much time to any one thing. This will also raise your dopamine and your acetylcholine levels.

- Meet new people. Start conversations when you usually would not. Do not wait for someone else to initiate one. Making new acquaintances raises your dopamine and GABA levels.

- Try communicating a different way. Introverts tend to process ideas internally and then put them into words. Start a dialogue that will allow you not only to relate your ideas as you process them but to share your feelings as well. This type of communication is good for your dopamine and your acetylcholine levels.

REACHING INTROVERT COMPETENCE

For an extrovert to become a little more introverted, you need to work on focus, paying attention to others, and silence. When you do so, you are learning how to turn off dopamine and direct your energy inward. At the same time, you will be raising your other biochemical levels.

- Try working on one thing at a time. See if you can work alone, quietly, without interruptions, giving yourself the time and space to do so. This activity will raise your acetylcholine levels and decrease dopamine.

- Spend time with a close friend. Listen to what he or she has to say before you share your thoughts. Think before you speak: complete your thoughts before you share them. Take the time to observe facial expressions and body language. This will raise both acetylcholine and serotonin levels, and diminish dopamine dominance.

- Do not let stress get to you. If you cannot handle a situation at the moment, then get away from it. Give yourself some time alone, whether it be to reflect or just time to cool down, then come back and solve the problem. This will raise both GABA and serotonin levels and diminish dopamine dominance.

BECOMING MORE SENSITIVE

For an intuitive acetylcholine nature to become a little more present, you have to become more detail-oriented, know the facts, and live in the present. When you are learning sensing competence, you are learning how to turn on your serotonin levels. Serotonin controls the feeling side of life. When we release serotonin we feel things more intensely. This is how you achieve true empathy.

- Prepare a special meal for yourself and a friend. Cook a new dish. Make sure to follow the recipe step by step. This will lower your acetylcholine and increase your serotonin and GABA levels.

- When you have a decision to make, sit down with a paper and pencil and list all the pros and cons of each choice. Then review your list, eliminating any assumptions you may have made along the way, focusing only on the actual facts in order to make your decision. This will lower your acetylcholine and increase your GABA levels.

- Review the chanting meditation in Chapter 7 before you go to sleep. Take ten minutes to reboot your brain by following this meditation. See if you get a better night's sleep and feel more

refreshed in the morning. Meditation will raise your serotonin
levels.

BECOMING MORE INTUITIVE

For a sensing nature to become a little more intuitive, you have to be creative and see the bigger picture. When you are learning intuitive competence, you are learning how to turn on acetylcholine. Acetylcholine is
all about awareness and creativity.

- Look around your home and see how your furnishings relate
  to your personality type. What does the décor say about you?
  This exercise raises acetylcholine.

- Think about what your life would be like if money was never an
  issue. You could do anything you wanted, whenever you wanted,
  with whomever you wanted. How would you live your life? This
  exercise raises both acetylcholine and dopamine levels.

- When you first walk into a room, take a quick glance and then
  close your eyes. Identify five small objects that are in the room,
  open your eyes, and find them. Then close your eyes again and
  try to identify five large objects that set the atmosphere of the
  room. This exercise raises acetylcholine and lowers GABA levels.

INCREASING YOUR RATIONAL THINKING STYLE

For the feeling to become a little more thought-directed, you have to
know the facts, use logic, and prepare for consequences. When you are
learning thinking competence, you are learning to turn on the power
and logic of dopamine.

- When making an important decision, make it based on facts.
  Do not allow others to interfere with your decision as long as
  your decision is fair. This exercise raises both acetylcholine and
  dopamine levels.

- Try starting your sentences with "I know . . ." instead of "I
  feel . . ." Be able to back up your thoughts with facts. This exercise raises dopamine levels.

- Communicate critical comments when needed. Know that
  you are doing it not to hurt the individual but for his or her

benefit. Be open and direct about it. This exercise raises both acetylcholine and dopamine levels.

- When problem solving, try looking at cause and effect. List all the possible outcomes and choose the one with the least negative outcomes. This exercise raises both acetylcholine and dopamine, and drops serotonin levels.

INCREASING YOUR FEELING THINKING STYLE

To become a little more feeling, you have to open up your heart. When you are learning feeling competence, you are learning how to turn on serotonin. Serotonin is all about feeling and pleasure.

- Listen, listen, and then listen a little more when people try to share their feelings with you. This exercise raises both acetyl-choline and serotonin levels.

- If you can help someone, do so, even if it means that you miss out on something. This exercise raises both acetylcholine and serotonin levels.

- Do not be afraid of saying "I love you" to others, even if they do not say it in return. This exercise raises dopamine and decreases serotonin.

JUDGING COMPETENCE

For a perceiver to become a little more judging, you need to plan ahead. Prioritizing and completing things in life are essential to make a change. When you are learning judging competence, you are learning to turn on GABA. GABA is all about balance.

- Make a list of activities that need to be accomplished, and pri-oritize them over an entire week. Work your way down the list using the weekend as your deadline. This exercise raises dopamine and lowers serotonin levels.

- Make sure that the essentials such as laundry and grocery shopping are done. Also, getting ready in the morning can go a lot smoother if you plan ahead. This exercise raises GABA and lowers serotonin levels.

PERCEIVING COMPETENCE

For a judging individual to become a little more perceiving, you need to become more flexible by being a knowledgeable risk taker. When you are learning perceiving competence, you are learning how to turn off GABA.

- Know your facts before you try to help someone out. It may be the difference between really good advice and poor advice. This exercise lowers your GABA levels.

- Do something you normally would not do. Return to a sport or hobby that you did as a child that was a lot of fun. This exercise lowers your GABA levels while raising your acetylcholine levels.

- Go out on the town with no plans, knowing that you're going to have fun. You do not always have to have an evening planned. This exercise lowers your GABA levels while raising your acetylcholine levels.

MANTRAS FOR THE NATURES

Here are some inspiring messages to help you with the above exercises. Using these mantras in combination with the exercises can help you find a more balanced mental state. Make it a habit to repeat these to yourself right before you go to bed at night, when you wake up in the morning, and throughout the day whenever relevant problems arise.

To Soften a Dopamine Nature
Whenever someone is trying to share an idea with me, I will listen to what he or she has to say.
I will learn not just to work with others but to work as a team player.
Whenever rules and regulations are implemented, I will try to understand their significance and follow them.
Whenever there is a task to complete, I will focus on the details so that it is completed to the best of my ability.

To Focus an Acetylcholine Nature

I will learn to understand the meaning behind the phrase "No one is perfect."

I will complete all my tasks, even the ones I wish someone else were doing.

Whenever a task becomes dull, I will stay focused and get the job done.

Whenever someone is making me a promise, I will trust that person and take that person at his or her word.

To Relax a GABA Nature

When I start to get tense, I will look at the big picture instead of focusing on the details.

Whenever I feel pain about others not doing things the right way, I need to take a step back and let others try their best. Only then will others see my good heart.

I must be patient when things do not go the way I expect them to.

To Strengthen a Serotonin Nature

I will try to have a little sensitivity toward others and not just think about myself.

I will assert my place in this world and ask for things that I need.

I have the strength to be responsible for my actions.

OVERCOMING THE DARK SIDE

The dark sides of our personalities are also driven by primary biochemicals. These aspects often occur as an excess or deficit in your particular nature. If you are experiencing any of the following negative personality traits and would like to do something in order to stop these behaviors, look to increase the biochemical that is most opposite to your nature.

Sometimes your dark side can work to your advantage. For example, it is normal to have loner tendencies as we grow older, due to hormonal loss that will create a dopamine deficiency. However, when our natures go out of whack, each strength of a personality becomes a weakness.

The following text lists each of the personality types and how these personalities can be bent through biochemistry. You can win the battle against your dark side by recognizing which biochemical needs to be enhanced and by following the treatment modalities listed in the nature chapters. Start by making small lifestyle and environment changes. You'll see results just by changing your diet and taking nutrient supplements. However, if you or others close to you feel that your behaviors are far from normal, you might need to seek psychiatric counseling.

Always keep in mind that that there are no pure personalities. We are all a mixture of many of these types. For example, at least 10 percent of all people have a little Loner in them, and 50 to 75 percent have traits of the Drama Queen. Most men (50 to 75 percent) are Self-Absorbed personalities, Rule Breakers, Dukes-Up types, or Perfectionists. Women, much more than men, usually have a Nurturing, sensitive streak. Between 5 and 10 percent of women have Abuse-Me personality components.

THE LONER

Normally this type is organized, neat, frugal, and no trouble to others. At its worst, it is as if this personality were born without feelings, incapable of experiencing strong emotions such as love, desire, joy, sadness, and rage. Loners talk and act with little animation, conveying a general monotony to the world. Given their natural remoteness, they prefer to be in the background, avoiding center stage until they reach their breaking point. In order to counteract this behavior, loners need to decrease their GABA and increase their dopamine so that they feel more assertive and have the confidence to get out into the world. Extreme loners have to be treated with dopamine stimulants.

PAINFULLY SHY

Normally this individual is sensitive to others, polite, caring, sweet, and sure not to offend anyone. At worst, this person is a walking social phobia: hesitant, distracted, edgy, vulnerable to any manner of criticism, and so morbidly afraid of being disliked that leading a lonely and empty life seems preferable. The painfully shy person sees himself as inadequate and inferior, which causes him to dismiss whatever success comes to him. He tends to live in the past and seek refuge in a fantasy world, where he can enjoy high self-esteem at will. In order to break this behavior, those who are painfully shy need to decrease their serotonin and increase their GABA, so that they can feel grounded in the real world. Painfully shy personalities frequently end up on serotonin-enhancing drugs such as Paxil, and anti-anxiety medications for their bashful natures.

THE NURTURING TYPE

Normally nurturers are caring, giving to others, needing others' approval, self-sacrificing, and passive decision makers who are tremendously involved in others' lives. At worst, these personalities spend their entire lives looking for love and opportunities to give care at the expense of being hurt when their own needs are not sufficiently met. They rely heavily on their mates and authority figures for advice—and can also fall into the trap of continuously craving and following the information of their peers. In order for nurturers to learn to let go of the responsibility of taking care of others, they need to decrease their GABA and increase dopamine. In this way they will begin to look out for themselves.

THE DRAMA QUEEN

Normally this type is a catalyst for creating change, growth, and development of self and others. At their worst they are theatrical to the max. Drama queens love and live for the big moment. They have a wild streak combined with a flirtatiousness that can often get them in hot water. This dark side can emerge in almost anyone during periods of high anxiety, when thinking confusion, trouble calculating, backaches, headaches, sweating, shaking, and palpitations will occur. If you are experiencing an intense need to be helped by others without helping yourself, you need to lower your dopamine levels and increase your GABA. Drama queens usually need leveling, so they often take anticonvulsants and other GABA-boosting agents.

SELF-ABSORBED

Normally this type is a high achiever. At worst, this personality profile is the epitome of the snob. Flouting conventional values as beneath them, they see themselves as entitled to make their own rules and let others be damned. Rationalization is part of the self-absorbed dark side. If you are feeling left behind by your friends or family, you might consider lowering your dopamine levels and increasing your serotonin. Then take a good look at how you've been treating others lately.

THE RULE BREAKER

Iconoclasts do not follow the group. They are shrewd operators, able to work around the rules of any system. At worst, they tend to be impulsive and shortsighted, proceeding rashly without considering the consequences of a deed. Personally irresponsible, they are given to insulting, even abusive actions about which they feel little or no remorse or guilt. They are intolerant and scornful of others. To get back into the good graces of the rest of society, rule breakers need to learn how to conform and mellow out by decreasing their dopamine and increasing their GABA.

DUKES-UP PERSONALITY

Normally this profile is intense, entrepreneurial, ambitious, challenging, and overachieving. However, this personality lashes out at others at the drop of a hat and can be verbally and physically abusive. Their memories are virtually all negative, heavy with a sense of injustice and the firm belief that the world has given them a raw deal. It's very hard for this personality type to get along with others because of the enormous chip on their shoulder. If this description fits you, you might want to decrease your dopamine and increase your GABA in order to get some balance and a more rational perspective on life.

THE PERFECTIONIST

Perfectionists are normally hardworking, detail-oriented, devoted, and exacting, all positive traits. However, the need for perfection can interfere with decision making, since striving for the ideal in everything is simply not realistic. These people are classic, active workaholics who retain tight self-control at the expense of relaxation, enjoyment, and warmth. If you are growing tired of this overwhelming need to control, you can decrease your GABA and increase your acetylcholine. This will give you a fresh, creative approach to problem solving, including the opportunity to delegate. Perfectionist personalities can also find themselves on medication and are frequently referred to therapists.

PROCRASTINATORS

We all can identify with procrastinators. However, their dark side is anger mixed with an avoidance of direct confrontation. In order to face life's challenges headfirst, procrastinators need to lower their serotonin and increase their acetylcholine.

THE ABUSE-ME PERSONALITY

Normally this profile is completely self-sacrificing for themselves and for the group. At worst, they find it almost impossible to experience joy and pleasure. Generally shy and retiring, someone with an abuse-me personality is more comfortable in a losing situation than a winning one. Interestingly, the deepest-feeling people have the lowest self-esteem. They are permitting themselves to shut off their own identity completely. That results in actively seeking condemnation and failing to accept whatever praise or support is offered—and deserved. If you feel this way, you need to beef up your own self-image by decreasing your serotonin and increasing your GABA. Abuse-me personalities often have extreme dopamine deficiencies that require medication.

ECCENTRICS

Eccentrics usually keep to themselves. At worst, they exhibit odd, even bizarre behavior. These personalities feel normal in isolated situations and steer away from human interaction. They live in a dream world composed of magical behavior and wild visions, although outwardly they appear colorless and inexpressive. When even mildly stressed, they can easily become a danger to others and themselves. Eccentrics need to decrease their serotonin and increase their dopamine in order to function outside of their own fantasy world.

THE UNSTABLE PERSONALITY

People with an unstable personality lack balance in all areas of life. They tend to bounce between extremes—from loving someone to hating him at the drop of a hat, from happiness to rage, and from being exercise fanatics to becoming bingers and substance abusers. They tend to neglect themselves and can never escape feelings of emptiness, which may be because of their ever-changing goals, friends, extracurricular activities, and values. Unstable personalities usually require significant psychiatric medications that will lower their dopamine levels while increasing their GABA.

THE SUSPICIOUS PERSONALITY

Suspicious personalities are hypervigilant. They are consummately skeptical, believing that everyone is out to get them. Rigid in ideology and reluctant to put trust in others, they tend to be loners, keeping their own skewed counsel at the cost of personal happiness. If your suspicious nature is taking over your life to the point where you are constantly worrying about those around you, consider lowering your dopamine and increasing your serotonin level.

EVERYBODY GETS ANXIOUS

On top of minor deficiencies, any one of us can experience brain chemistry problems when we are feeling anxious or depressed. Anxiety begins the entire health slide to the darker aspects of your personality and can affect different personalities in different ways. With increased anxiety, a Rule Breaker can become absolutely fierce. Add the blues to a Drama Queen, and she tries to avoid everything. Anxiety will make a Self-Absorbed person feel ashamed or furious. A depressed Abuse-Me type will crawl into a corner and hide. Once again, the good news is that we can target the disturbance at the source—the brain itself.

If you can learn to distinguish the early warning signs of anxiety and depression, you can stop your personality from sliding into total darkness. For example, many of us can sense when we are not quite feeling like ourselves. During these periods, we are actually struggling with our dark sides. If you can recognize when your personality is starting to slip, and follow the nutrient programs of the opposite nature, you can regain a balanced brain. In times of overwhelming anxiety, seek professional medical attention for the proper medications that can address your condition.

I have also found that depression exacerbates most physical illnesses. Even with the more serious diseases such as Alzheimer's and hypertension, most of my patients see direct physical benefits from taking antidepressants. Talk to your physician about including antidepressants in your medication regimen. If you inform your doctor of the results of your Braverman Nature Assessment, he or she will be able to prescribe the right medication that matches your nature as well as your symptoms.

MASTERING THE EDGE EFFECT

You now have at your disposal a complete program for reaching your full mental potential. You can decide to remedy a personality deficiency or increase all of your chemistry to achieve the four aspects of the edge. You can pick and choose what you want to change about your personality depending on the direction you would like to see your life going, or even to accomplish a single task. You can increase your dopamine whenever you need extra power, increase your acetylcholine if you want to achieve higher consciousness, increase your GABA to get to the Zen state of ultimate calm, or raise your serotonin whenever you feel overloaded with information, so that your brain can reboot over a good night's sleep.

Whatever you decide is right for you, as long as you understand your nature as well as your treatment options. With this knowledge, you can enjoy the full benefits of the Edge Effect.

12

MASTERING THE EDGE EFFECT

FOR LASTING HEALTH

By READING THIS book, you have taken the first important step toward achieving total physical and mental health. You now have at your disposal a complete program that explains how the brain controls the body's functions and how you can adjust and even augment its capabilities. Specifically, you've learned that by improving your brain chemistry you can enhance your nature and address your deficiencies. In doing so, you will improve your physical health and mental well-being; you'll be a beneficiary of the Edge Effect.

FOLLOWING THE BRAVERMAN
PRESCRIPTION

There is much to achieve by following this program: once you've identified your own brain-dominant nature and identified any imbalances, the opportunities for improving your physical and mental self are limitless. If you find your brain is in balance and that you are symptom-free, you can choose to work on whatever aspect of your present life deserves focus. For example, you can adjust your brain chemistry to achieve weight loss, enjoy more fulfilling sexual experiences, and even modify your temperament. As long as you understand your nature and your treatment options, you can use the Edge Effect to become a better, healthier person.

You can learn to recognize the merits of each nature and incorporate their best traits into your own. For example, if you haven't been sleeping well, you can boost your serotonin for almost instant results. Or, if you need to stay up late to finish a report, you'll know how to boost you dopamine level for more energy. By enhancing your biochemical combination as you see fit, you will begin to experience what I call the Ultimate Edge Effect, where your mind and body perform at optimal levels of efficiency. Whichever path you choose to bring you to greater mental, physical, and spiritual wellness, they all begin with the same simple steps.

First, take the Braverman Nature Assessment. By taking this test, you will discover your true biochemical nature and become aware of any deficiencies or excesses. With this knowledge, you become an educated consumer in the world of health care. You will be able to intelligently discuss with your doctor not only what your symptoms are but what you believe might be causing them. Remember, most illnesses can be directly related to brain chemical imbalances.

The adjustment to better health requires work. My program is only as good as the effort you put into it. Even when you are feeling well, you need to periodically retest your brain balance. I recommend that you should take the Braverman Nature Assessment at least three times each year. Your results will change each time, depending on your physical and mental well-being. Each time, you will be able to create a new strategy for improving yourself and your overall health.

The next step is to address your deficiencies. If you are experiencing specific illnesses or ailments, you will find significant relief once you regain brain balance and have recovered your edge. Remember, achieving brain balance and total wellness does not always occur instantaneously. Depending on which treatment options you choose or the severity of your illness, you might experience incremental, rather than instant, relief. If you are experiencing minor brain nature-related symptoms, you should follow the personalized treatment program, which includes changes to your environment, lifestyle, and diet that support your brain-dominant nature. If you have moderate or severe symptoms, you should work with your physician to create a prescription regimen using nature-specific medications and natural hormones to get your health back on track. Once you begin following these guidelines, you will quickly find that enhancing your brain chemistry will become second nature. More important, your ailments will melt away, and serious illnesses can recede. Never give up hope: you can feel better again.

Now, focus on making the most of your primary nature. When you feel physically and mentally comfortable, you have successfully balanced your own nature and have begun to experience the Edge Effect. You might feel a variety of new sensations, depending on your nature. If you are a dopamine nature, you might feel the metabolic high of intensity, what I like to call "the zone," which leads to a healthy, fit, energetic body. An acetylcholine nature can reach an enthusiastic state of higher consciousness, where you might uncover your artistic or spiritual side. Or a GABA nature can have a Zen experience, becoming an even more stable, even-keeled, and organized person. Serotonin natures can learn to reboot their brain by boosting serotonin, reaching a calmness that is the natural result of serenity.

Lastly, use the Edge Effect to experience higher performance in ways you never imagined possible. Once you master your nature, you can try for the ultimate edge, where total health—mental, physical, and spiritual—is achieved along with a longer, richer, and more satisfying life. We're all getting older, but how we experience the later years of our lives is completely in our hands. This book has taught you to recognize how your body ages and how you can keep yourself one step ahead of nature's plan. When you maintain proper brain chemistry, you can postpone the pauses that contribute to aging as well as the myriad diseases that are caused by even the most minor biochemical failures. By taking care of your brain and body today through proper nutrition, good lifestyle choices, and, when necessary, medication, you may be preventing a lifetime of illness.

What's more, a healthy and supple brain is necessary for memory retention. Following an acetylcholine-boosting program is the most important thing you can do to preserve, and possibly enhance, your memory capabilities. The Braverman Memory Test can help you uncover any possible issue regarding your memory or cognitive failure. If you have discovered a minor deficiency, you can begin to treat yourself with brain exercises that improve working, immediate, verbal, and visual memory. If you have discovered a moderate or severe deficiency, you can inform your doctor of your test scores and together you can create an aggressive campaign of supplements (and possibly medication) to stop the damage from progressing, so that you will be able to enjoy a sound mind through your old age.

With both your body and brain functioning at peak performance, all that prevents you from experiencing true happiness is yourself. Luckily, you now have the ability to modify your personality by fine-tuning your brain chemistry. Done properly, you can affect lasting changes to your temperament and modify your day-to-day character in order to feel more comfortable with yourself and others. In this way, bending your personality through biochemistry can help you learn to love—and be loved—more completely.

You can choose what you want to change about your personality whether you are looking for permanent change in your life or need to make a minor adjustment in order to more efficiently accomplish a single task. For example, you can increase your dopamine when you need to be a little more forceful, increase your acetylcholine if you want to become more thoughtful, or increase your GABA to tone down your anxieties. Finally, you can increase your serotonin when you need to be more social.

GETTING FROM THE BALANCED BRAIN TO THE ULTIMATE EDGE EFFECT

When you have done the work on all four corners of the edge, you have successfully learned to bend your brain to take your personality, temperament, and physical body to a superior state—the Ultimate Edge Effect. By reaching this state, you have effectively decoded the brain's impact on your health. All of your four primary neurotransmitters are at their peak levels, creating the ultimate brain-mind-body connection. When this happens, your mind and body are working better than ever, and you will experience moments of transcendent joy and oneness with all things.

The Ultimate Edge Effect includes optimum dopamine-zone metabolism: you are flying, racing, doing a million things with total clarity and purpose. Simultaneously, you are in a state of acetylcholine nirvana, where you can be loving, giving, and empathetic to others. Your GABA outward calm does not give way to your intensity. And at night, you reach complete serotonin serenity as your sleep is deep and sound, with your mind open and accepting of your unconscious dream state. This is the time when your brain will process and purge excess information, leaving you refreshed and renewed the next day.

I have been fortunate enough to reach this Ultimate Edge in my life. At these moments I have felt more than just physical and mental peace, and it is a feeling beyond words. I know that you can enjoy this remarkable experience as well. If you are open to the challenges of this program, then you can reach this Ultimate Edge, and more.

TOWARD A BETTER FUTURE

In my office I see miracles happen every day. I know that this program works, that miracles are real, and that anyone can benefit from my program, no matter how they feel today. Your ability to understand how the brain functions and how it impacts the entire mind and body will determine how you use this information. I hope you have found, as I have, that the brain is more than just another one of your internal organs; it holds the secret to a better, fuller life, which, when revealed, can change the way you live every day and forever.

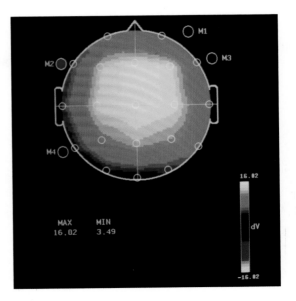

A healthy BEAM Image. This brain shows a large yellow burst in the center of the brain, with strong, balanced color spread evenly throughout the entire brain. This brain is functioning at 16 micro volts of energy and at a P300 speed of 280.

P300=280ms

INTRODUCTION TO BEAM: THE BEAM™

The most reliable test of brain function is the Brain Electrical Activity Map, or BEAM™. First developed by researchers at Harvard Medical School in the 1980s, this computer-based technique measures the electrical activity of the brain.

The BEAM assesses the brain's electrical transmissions by measuring the four individual brain waves and brain-wave combinations. This provides an accurate graphic depiction of the four primary brain biochemicals. Once a treatment program is underway, we can accurately assess its effectiveness.

The first measure of brain health is voltage, which determines the brain's electrical power and is an associated with the biochemical dopamine. In the photograph above, the yellow center flowing into strong red colors indicates high energy. This brain is operating at a high voltage of 16 micro volts, which is shown on the bar in the lower right corner.

The second measure of brain health is electrical speed, recorded in milliseconds. Brain speed is associated with the biochemical acetylcholine. Strong reds and yellow dominate the photograph above, indicators of both high energy and quick speed. The P300 value, which is a measure of brain speed, is 280 milliseconds, as indicated in the caption.

The third measure of brain health is rhythm. Rhythm is associated with the biochemical GABA. In the photograph above, the electrical wave patterns indicate accurate rhythm; the yellow and red colors are evenly spread throughout the BEAM image.

The last measure of brain health is synchrony, or wave balance between hemispheres controlled by seratonin. The photograph above shows wave patterns emanating from the brain's center with beautiful symmetry into the right and left hemispheres and the front and rear lobes. This indicates good communication between both the right and left hemispheres and all lobes of the brain.

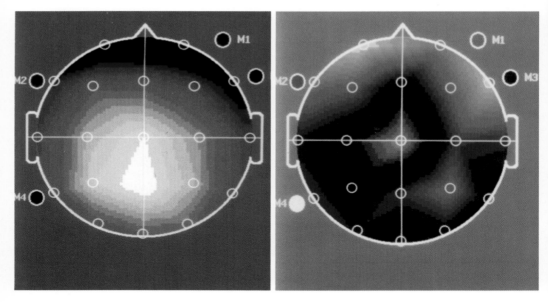

Healthy Dopamine Brain   *Unbalanced Dopamine Brain*

DOPAMINE BEAM

The photograph on the left shows a normal, healthy dopamine balanced brain. The bright yellows and reds indicate high energy, and the voltage level measures 10 micro volts. The right image shows a near absence of yellow-red color—only a small burst of red appears in the center of the brain—with black and dark blue dominant overall. The black indicates virtually no dopamine activity with slight activity showing as dark blue. The voltage level in the photograph on the right is extremely low and measures 2 micro volts. This is a picture of a brain with very low energy. Obesity is associated with a dopamine deficiency. When the brain lacks energy, the body's metabolism is low and it cannot process food efficiently. The body compensates by demanding more food, which provides short term energy, but unless the brain gets the dopamine it needs, the body will continue to expand as energy continues to diminish.

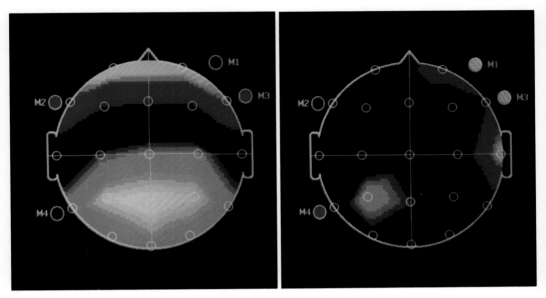

Healthy Acetylcholine Brain   *Unbalanced Acetylcholine Brain*

ACETYLCHOLINE BEAM

A major acetylcholine deficiency will be evident by a high P300 score. The photograph on the left shows a brain with a normal balance of acetylcholine. The P300 reading is 290 milliseconds and there are intense yellows and reds, indicators of high brain processing speed, commonly associated with "quick thinking." The photograph on the right indicates an acetylcholine deficiency with a P300 reading of 390 milliseconds. The absence of yellow and the small isolated burst of dull red indicate extremely low acetylcholine levels and a very slow, seriously troubled brain. A P300 score higher than 300 milliseconds indicates a decline in brain speed, which becomes more and more significant as speed drops. Declining speed affects our memory and thinking ability; slow brain speed can be an early warning sign of Alzheimer's disease.

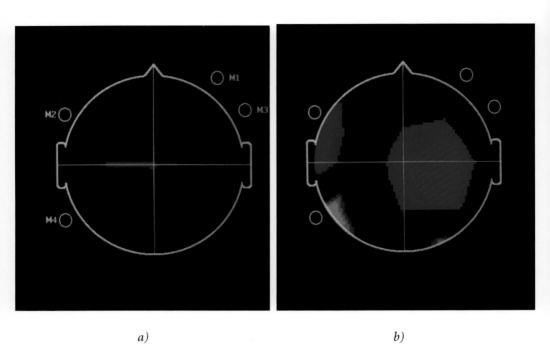

a)   b)

Varying Degrees of GABA deficiency from mild to severe.

GABA BEAM

The BEAM is particularly effective to visually demonstrate a GABA deficiency. Each of the wave patterns, shown from left to right, display increasing disruptions in rhythmic wave function. Deviation in brain rhythms manifest as being too fast or to slow, too excitable or too dull. You can see that the over-all color shifts from a stable black-blue background to increasing amounts and intensities of light blue, demonstrating brain-wave rhythm disorders caused by decreasing GABA levels. Photograph (a) indicates normal GABA levels and good brain rhythm function. Photograph (b) demonstrates minor rhythm disturbances such as you might find in a patient with allergies. Photograph (c) shows a patient with moderate GABA deficiency who might be experiencing various anxiety-related symptoms, a faster than normal pulse rate, and high blood pressure. Photograph (d) indicates a severe GABA imbalance and might manifest, along with the other GABA deficient symptoms, as short-tempered raging.

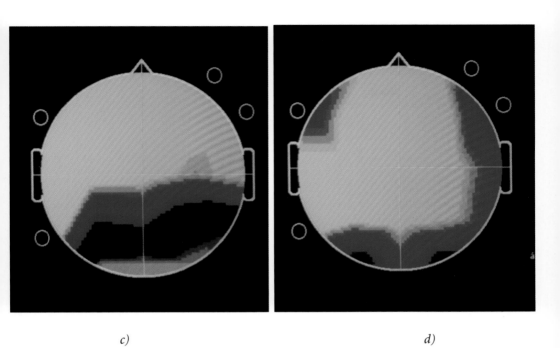

c)   d)

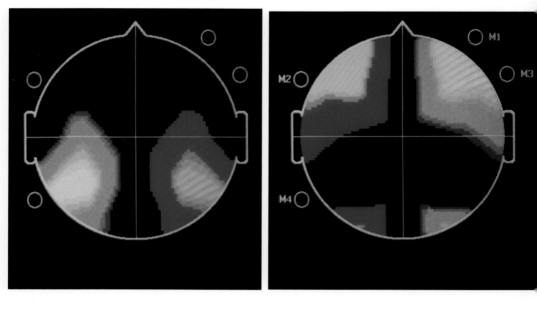

a)   b)

Varying Degrees of serotonin deficiency from mild to severe.

SEROTONIN BEAM

Serotonin deficiency appears as wave pattern imbalances between the brain's hemispheres and/or lobes. In each of the photographs above, notice the color asymmetry between the right and left hemispheres. In each photograph one side of the brain shows a predominant red hue, while the other hemisphere is blue, indicating a left-right brain imbalance. The enlarging of the color areas demonstrates increasing levels of serotonin deficiency. Photograph (a) shows a mild serotonin imbalance, typical of PMS in women or premature ejaculation in men. Photograph (b) indicates a mild abnormality in symmetry and is commonly seen associated with irritable bowel syndrome. Photograph (c) demonstrates numerous moderate serotonin imbalances typical of a wide range of disorders including perimenopausal symptoms and mood disorders. Photograph (d) illustrates a severe serotonin imbalance, particularly in the frontal lobes. This is typical with excitable, emotional individuals with severe insomnia.

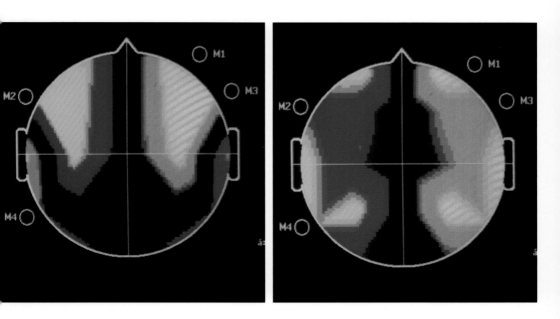

c)   *d)*

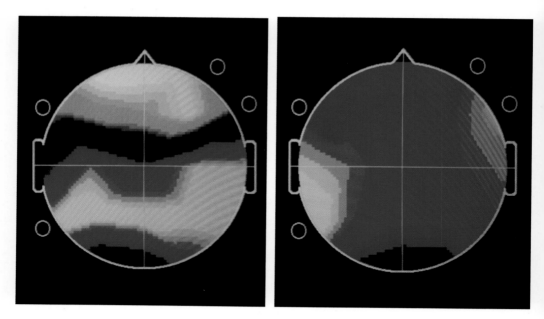

*a) BEAM scan of a patient
with an aged brain.*

*b) BEAM scan of same patient
after treatment.*

THE EDGE EFFECT

The two photographs show how dramatic the results of The Edge Effect program can be. In this case, a 40-year-old woman came to me suffering from short-term memory problems, obesity, a sense of disorganization, and sleep disorders. She felt constantly fatigued, had no energy, and was unable to think clearly and quickly. She had been to a number of other doctors, each of whom prescribed various drugs that treated her symptoms, but her symptoms kept getting worse. The first step for this patient was getting a BEAM. The BEAM scan (photograph a) shows what her brain looked like during her first visit. The BEAM shows clear signs of premature aging: low dopamine levels (voltage registered as 0.5) and severely low levels of acetylcholine (P300 = 375), as well as indicators of GABA deficiencies and serotonin imbalances. We developed a diet, drug program, changes to both her lifestyle and environment, and a promise on her part to adhere to this program and return to my office for regular check-ups.

Nine months later, a bright, trim, confident, and energetic woman walked into my office. Her last BEAM scan (photograph b) shows almost full recovery. Her voltage levels were now at a normal 10, her P300 reading was a normal 320, and both her GABA and serotonin levels indicated greatly improved brain rhythm and synchrony. She had restored her Edge. The balanced patient is now intense, enthusiastic, organized, and calm. Her brain, mind, and body health have been fully restored.

INDEX